WORKBOOK TO ACCOMPANY

The Basic EMT
COMPREHENSIVE PREHOSPITAL PATIENT CARE

Norman E. McSwain, Jr., M.D., F.A.C.S.
Professor of Surgery
Tulane University School of Medicine
New Orleans, LA

Roger D. White, M.D., F.A.C.S.
Professor of Anesthesiology
Mayo Clinic
Rochester, MN

James L. Paturas, EMT-P
Director, Emergency Medical Services
Bridgeport Hospital
Bridgeport, CT

William R. Metcalf, EMT-B
EMS Executive Officer
North Lake Tahoe Fire District
Lake Tahoe, NV

CHIEF EDITOR: Brenda J. Beasley, RN, BS, EMT-Paramedic

Editor: Michael J. Thornton, NREMT-P

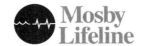

Mosby Lifeline

St. Louis Baltimore Boston Carlsbad Chicago Naples New York Philadelphia Portland
London Madrid Mexico City Singapore Sydney Tokyo Toronto Wiesbaden

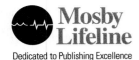
Mosby
Lifeline
Dedicated to Publishing Excellence

A Times Mirror
Company

Senior Vice President: David T. Culverwell
Publisher: David Dusthimer
Executive Editor: Claire Merrick
Editor: Julie Scardiglia
Assistant Editors: Lisa Benson, John Goucher
Developmental Editor: Kathleen Scogna
Editorial Assistant: Sheri Fentress
Project Manager: Chris Baumle
Production Editor: David Orzechowski
Designer: Nancy McDonald
Cover Design: Ox and Company

Printed in the United States of America
Composition by Digitype
Printed by Plus Communications

Mosby–Year Book, Inc.
11830 Westline Industrial Drive
St. Louis, Missouri 63146

ISBN 0-8151-5979-X

97 98 99 00 01/9 8 7 6 5 4 3

This Workbook that accompanies *The Basic EMT: Comprehensive Prehospital Patient Care* is designed to help you, the student, master the skills and knowledge necessary to become a successful EMT-Basic. A diligent effort to complete each chapter of this workbook will not only help you remember and retain the skills and knowledge presented in the EMT-Basic course, but will guide you in applying your newly-acquired knowledge to typical situations encountered in the prehospital environment.

Each Workbook chapter is keyed to chapters in *The Basic EMT: Comprehensive Prehospital Patient Care*. To make the most of your EMT training, it is suggested that you read each textbook chapter thoroughly and answer the review questions found at the back of each chapter. Then, complete the Workbook exercises for that chapter and check your answers. If you have answered a question incorrectly, go back and review that section of the textbook chapter. After you have reviewed the section, attempt to answer the Workbook question again. With this strategy of review and attention, you should easily overcome areas of difficulty.

Each chapter of the Workbook has the following sections:

- A list of the chapter objectives found in *The Basic EMT: Comprehensive Prehospital Patient Care.*

- An Introduction that summarizes the key points of the chapter content.

- Review questions in true/false, fill-in-the-blank, and multiple choice formats. Each review question is keyed to a text objective.

- Answers to the review questions.

- One or more scenarios that present an example of an EMS situation appropriate to the chapter content. Students are asked to apply the skills and knowledge learned in the textbook in order to demonstrate the correct assessment and management of a typical patient.

- Solutions to the scenarios so that students can check their answers.

It is hoped that this Workbook will become an integral part of your EMT-Basic education. Good luck with the course and with your future career in EMS.

This book is dedicated in loving memory of my father,

W. Jack Messer, who was always there for me,

and in honor of my dear friend and mentor,

Dr. Willis D. Israel,

who is responsible for my venture into EMS.

BJB

CONTENTS

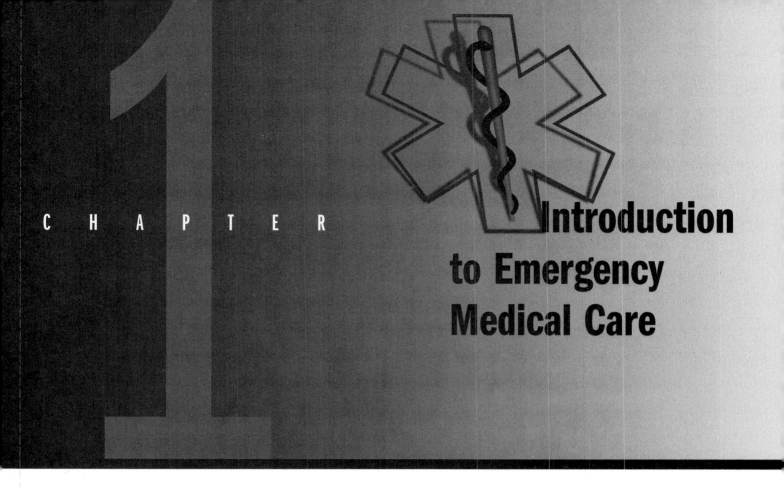

CHAPTER 1

Introduction to Emergency Medical Care

Reading Assignment: Chapter 1, pgs. 1–16

OBJECTIVES

1. Define emergency medical care.

2. Explain how emergency medical care relates to other components of the healthcare delivery system.

3. Define the role that emergency medical services play in the public health community and in the public safety community.

4. Define Emergency Medical Technician (EMT).

5. Describe pertinent history, current events, and the future outlook for the EMT.

6. Identify the role played by the U.S. Department of Transportation in the training of the EMT.

7. Describe the difference between an assessment-based approach to emergency care and a diagnoses-based approach.

8. Explain the differing goals of initial and continuing education for the EMT.

9. Identify the various components of EMT training.

10. Identify the various certifying bodies for the EMT.

INTRODUCTION

Emergency medical care describes care rendered to those who become seriously ill or injured. It entails rapid response, assessment, stabilization, transportation, and definitive care. The EMT is a vital component of the emergency medical care system.

The core content of this book is directed towards presenting the knowledge base necessary to be an effective EMT-B. The EMT-B is the heart of the emergency medical care system.

REVIEW QUESTIONS

Please circle one correct answer for each question.

1. The general term used to describe medical care that is provided to people who suddenly become seriously ill or injured is: (C 1-1.1)
   a. triage
   b. definitive care
   c. acute care services
   d. emergency medical care

2. The process of determining the nature and extent of the patient's illness or injury is called: (C 1-1.1)
   a. stabilization
   b. assessment
   c. diagnosis
   d. prognosis

3. A well-organized Emergency Medical Services (EMS) system is capable of meeting all the potential healthcare needs of the community. (C 1-1.2)
   a. true
   b. false

4. Services provided by society to meet the basic needs of the population are known as: (C 1-1.7)
   a. statutes
   b. utilities
   c. public safety services
   d. health maintenance organizations

5. The heart of the EMS system is the: (C 1-1.2)
   a. physician
   b. first responder
   c. EMT
   d. EMS dispatcher

6. At the national level, there are _____ levels of EMT. (C 1-1.2)
   a. 4
   b. 2
   c. 5
   d. 3

7. The term used to describe the basic level of EMT training developed by the U.S. Department of Transportation is: (C 1-1.2)

    a. FIRST RESPONDER
    b. EMT-Intermediate
    c. EMT-Paramedic
    d. EMT-B

8. The 1966 research paper, which strongly recommends that a standard defining the minimum level of training for prehospital providers be established, is: (C 1-1.1)

    a. Medical Practice Act
    b. U.S. Constitution
    c. Accidental Death and Disability: The Neglected Disease of Modern Society
    d. Harrison Narcotic Act: Food, Drug and Cosmetic Act of 1966

9. Responsibility for the development of training programs for prehospital providers is assigned to: (C 1-1.1)

    a. U.S. Department of Defense
    b. U.S. Department of Health Care
    c. U.S. Department of Transportation
    d. U.S. Department of Management and Finance

10. Legislation enacted in 1973 that set the stage for standardized training of prehospital personnel is called the: (C 1-1.1)

    a. Emergency Medical Services System Act
    b. National Highway Traffic Safety Act
    c. Department of Transportation Act
    d. Medical Practice Act

11. The primary purpose of continuing education for the EMT is: (C 1-1.7)

    a. to teach new information
    b. to provide quality patient care
    c. to enhance financial security
    d. to enhance job security

12. The initial responsibility of the EMT at the scene with an ill or injured patient is to assure: (C 1-1.3)

    a. scene safety
    b. traffic control
    c. rapid treatment
    d. rapid transport

13. Patient care based on a simple recognition of the patient's signs and symptoms is referred to as (a/an): (C 1-1.2)

    a. overview of the scene
    b. diagnoses-based approach
    c. assessment-based approach
    d. definitive medical care approach

14. In the initial phase of the EMS educational process, the basic knowledge and skills necessary to be fully functional in the prehospital setting are emphasized. (C 1-1.2)

    a. true
    b. false

15. A prerequisite for entrance into the EMT-B training program is: (C 1-1.1)

    a. ARC
    b. CPR
    c. EVO
    d. BSI

16. A national, nonprofit registration agency for prehospital providers that uses a written examination and a skills competency practical examination is the: (C 1-1.7)

    a. National Academy of Health Sciences
    b. National Registry of Emergency Medical Technicians
    c. National Association of Emergency Medical Technicians
    d. American Medical Association

17. A clinical experience is one that provides the student with the opportunity to practice patient assessment and skills on actual patients. (C 1-1.1)

    a. true
    b. false

18. The EMT-B training program involves at least ＿＿ hours of classroom instruction plus clinical experience.

    a. 80
    b. 100
    c. 200
    d. 110

19. The EMT-B training course requires a commitment from the student to study outside the classroom in order to adequately comprehend the curriculum content.

    a. true
    b. false

20. In the future, EMTs will be involved in research that will include patient data entry and analysis.

    a. true
    b. false

Scenarios

Read each scenario. Write the answers to the corresponding questions in the space provided.

SCENARIO #1:

Today is the first day of your EMT-B course. You are en route to the local community college where the training program is conducted. Approximately one mile from the college, you witness a single car veer off the road and strike a power pole. The car overturns and two victims are ejected from the vehicle.

You stop at the scene of the accident. One victim has a bluish discoloration of his skin. The other victim is lying face down and the only sound you hear resembles snoring. You notice gasoline pouring from the vehicle.

1. List at least two hazards present at the scene.

    gasoline, electrical wires, unstable vehicle, traffic

SCENARIO #2:

You have successfully completed the EMT-B education course and have been employed with a local ambulance service for four weeks. You and your partner, who is an EMT-Intermediate, are called to the scene of a diving accident at the city pool.

When you arrive on the scene, you note that the patient has been pulled from the pool and is lying by the side of the pool. The patient is unresponsive. Bystanders state that the patient struck his head when diving from the high board. When you approach the patient, you are informed that there are two nurses present. They are assessing the patient's vital signs.

1. As a newly graduated EMT-B, you realize that scene control and patient care should be managed by which healthcare professional?

    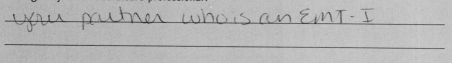
    your partner who is an EMT-I

2. How could the transition of care best be handled?

    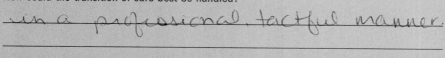
    in a professional, tactful manner.

CHAPTER 1 ANSWERS TO REVIEW QUESTIONS

4. c	8. c	12. a	16. b	20. a
3. b	7. d	11. b	15. b	19. a
2. b	6. d	10. a	14. a	18. d
1. d	5. c	9. c	13. c	17. a

CHAPTER 1 SCENARIOS SOLUTIONS

Scenario #1:

1. Hazards present at the scene are as follows:
   - gasoline
   - electrical wires
   - unstable vehicle
   - traffic

Scenario #2:

1. The scene should be managed by your partner, who is an EMT-Intermediate.
2. The transition should be handled in a professional, tactful manner.

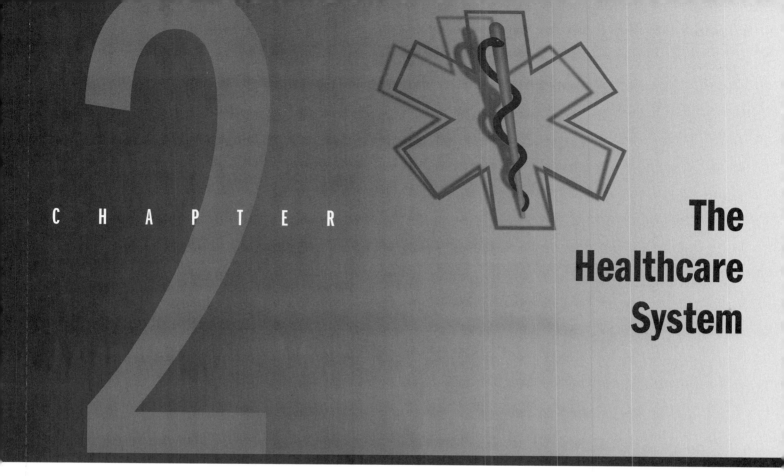

CHAPTER 2

The Healthcare System

Reading Assignment: Chapter 2, pgs. 17–27

OBJECTIVES

1. Demonstrate a basic understanding of the types of health care that are available in the United States.

2. Describe how the components of the healthcare system are integrated.

3. Explain how the EMS system interacts with the healthcare system.

4. Identify the changes occurring in the healthcare system.

5. Describe how changes in the healthcare system will affect the EMS system.

INTRODUCTION

The healthcare system in the United States functions through a partnership between governments (federal and state) and private providers. The government provides specific health and welfare programs for the elderly, the disabled, and the poor. These programs are known as Medicare and Medicaid.

The Medicare and Medicaid programs do not literally provide healthcare, but they supply insurance so that beneficiaries can have access to care. Private providers of care such as hospitals, health maintenance organizations (HMOs), physicians, and other allied health professionals offer the care necessary to the recipient of Medicare or Medicaid. Through this process, government and the private healthcare providers work in partnership.

This chapter discusses integrated healthcare delivery and how the different components of the system provide for a comprehensive approach. There is also a review of the relationship between the emergency medical system and the other components of healthcare. A mutual dependency exists between the emergency medical system and other aspects of the healthcare system.

▪ REVIEW QUESTIONS

Please circle one correct answer for each question.

1. The healthcare system in the United States operates through a partnership between government (federal and state) and private providers. (C 1-1.1)

   a. true
   b. false

2. Specific health and welfare programs are provided by the government for the elderly, the disabled, and the poor. One example of these programs is: (C 1-1.1)

   a. Medicare
   b. Gericare
   c. HMO
   d. Red Cross

3. Medicare is: (C 1-1.1)

   a. a program for minorities
   b. a health insurance program for the elderly
   c. a state mandated developmental program for the elderly
   d. a health management organizational plan

4. In certain instances, permanently disabled individuals are eligible for Medicare benefits even if they are less than 65 years of age. (C 1-1.1)

   a. true
   b. false

5. The Medicaid program: (C 1-1.1)

   a. provides health insurance to the poor regardless of age
   b. requires that an individual or family meet specific financial requirements for the poverty level
   c. does not actually provide healthcare, but does provide insurance so that beneficiaries can have access to care
   d. all of the above

6. The emergency medical system and other aspects of the healthcare system are mutually dependent. (C 1-1.1)

   a. true
   b. false

7. Emergency care provided outside the hospital that integrates with and supports the healthcare delivery system is known as the: (C 1-1.1)

   a. prehospital system
   b. medical services system
   c. emergency department services
   d. tertiary care services

8. Financing or payment for EMS care is most often provided through: (C 1-1.1)

   a. insurance
   b. managed care
   c. self-pay
   d. subscription

9. Acute care is the medical treatment provided in response to a medical condition of sudden onset and short duration intended to stabilize the patient's condition prior to moving on to definitive care. (C 1-1.1)

   a. true
   b. false

10. The treatment provided to cure or solve the patient's current illness or injury is known as: (C 1-1.1)

    a. preventive care
    b. postmortem care
    c. definitive care
    d. inpatient care

11. The acute care facility provides: (C 1-1.1)

    a. emergency and trauma care
    b. critical intensive care
    c. surgical intervention and diagnostic testing services
    d. all of the above

12. Restorative care involves the treatment and therapy necessary to return the patient to a "normal" condition or function. (C 1-1.1)

    a. true
    b. false

13. The focus in the healthcare system is: (C 1-1.1)

    a. community education
    b. for the patient to improve
    c. financial accountability
    d. governmental statutes and regulations

14. The type of care required when a patient continues to need healthcare intervention and does not improve is known as: (C 1-1.1)

    a. acute care
    b. ambulatory care
    c. preventive care
    d. chronic care

15. Chronic care is provided in locations such as: (C 1-1.1)

    a. extended care facilities
    b. nursing homes
    c. the patient's own home
    d. all of the above

16. Healthcare providers include: (C 1-1.1)

    a. EMT-B
    b. EMT-Paramedic
    c. physicians
    d. all of the above

17. EMTs provide: (C 1-1.2)

    a. initial assessment and stabilization
    b. transport of the patient
    c. physician delegated activities
    d. all of the above

18. The "captain of the ship" in the healthcare system is: (C 1-1.6)

    a. the physician
    b. the hospital administrator
    c. the chief of the local fire department
    d. the EMT-Paramedic

19. Types of nurses include: (C 1-1.1)

    a. all the below are correct
    b. licensed practical nurses
    c. licensed vocational nurses
    d. registered nurses

20. Dynamic forces are changing the healthcare system. The most significant is: (C 1-1.1)

    a. significant increases in the cost of healthcare
    b. government healthcare payers
    c. the consensus of politicians
    d. healthcare administrators

21. In the fee-for-service model, the patient: (C 1-1.1)

    a. accesses a health service
    b. pays a fee for such care
    c. provides a major focus on preventive care
    d. a and b are correct

22. In the managed care environment, physician providers, specialists, and provider organizations such as acute care facilities are preselected by the: (C 1-1.1)

    a. providers
    b. insurer
    c. patient
    d. community

23. With the capitation approach: (C 1-1.1)

    a. the fee is usually paid on an annual basis for the individuals covered under the insurance plan
    b. there is no set fee for the service provided to the patient
    c. the insurer pays for a specific menu of healthcare services at a fixed fee
    d. the patient pays the fee prior to treatment

24. One global change in the healthcare system is the shift from "fee-for-service" financing to "managed care." (C 1-1.1)

    a. true
    b. false

25. Many demands are placed on the prehospital provider in the managed care environment. The greatest demand is: (C 1-1.5)

    a. assuring for the delivery of appropriate care to the patient
    b. increasing scrutiny being placed on the health management organizations
    c. monitoring quality assurance
    d. financial accountability of the provider service

26. The managed care system focuses on: (C 1-1.1)

    a. public education
    b. insurance managers
    c. physician management
    d. preventive care

27. Preventive care includes: (C 1-1.1)

    a. health screening
    b. physical examinations
    c. immunizations
    d. all of the above

28. HMO is the abbreviation for: (C 1-1.1)

    a. home maintenance organization
    b. health maintenance organization
    c. health medical organization
    d. hospice medical objective

Scenarios

Read each scenario. Write the answers to the corresponding questions in the space provided.

SCENARIO #1:

You have responded to a call for help from an elderly male who is experiencing pains in his chest. Upon arrival at his home, his daughter meets you outside the residence stating that her father is retired. She asks whether "the government" will pay the ambulance bill for her father.

1. About which government insurance program is she inquiring?

medical

SCENARIO #2:

Your EMS organization is co-sponsoring the County Health Fair. You and your partner are in charge of blood pressure screening for the afternoon. You have been instructed by the EMS Medical Director that any patient with an abnormal blood pressure reading should be referred to his or her personal physician. The hospital association is offering free hearing and vision screening tests, as well as chest x-rays.

1. What type of care is being provided to these participants at the Health Fair?

preventative health care

CHAPTER 2 ANSWERS TO REVIEW QUESTIONS

1. a	**7.** a	**13.** b	**19.** a	**25.** a
2. a	**8.** a	**14.** d	**20.** a	**26.** d
3. b	**9.** a	**15.** d	**21.** d	**27.** d
4. a	**10.** c	**16.** d	**22.** b	**28.** b
5. d	**11.** d	**17.** d	**23.** c	
6. a	**12.** a	**18.** a	**24.** a	

SCENARIOS SOLUTIONS

Scenario #1:   1. Medicare

Scenario #2:   2. Preventive healthcare

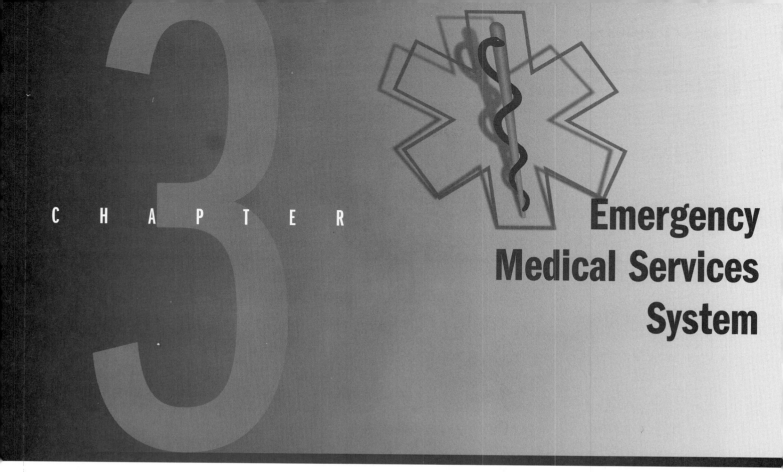

CHAPTER 3

Emergency Medical Services System

Reading Assignment: Chapter 3, pgs. 28–47

OBJECTIVES

1. Describe the EMS system and identify each of its component parts.

    - Regulation and policy
    - Resource management
    - Human resource and training
    - Transportation
    - Facilities
    - Communications
    - Public information and education
    - Medical direction
    - Trauma systems
    - Evaluation

2. Identify common EMS system models.

3. Describe current challenges facing EMS systems.

4. Identify current trends and potential changes in EMS systems.

▌ INTRODUCTION

The evolutionary process of the EMS system continues on a daily basis. The EMS system is an intricate arrangement that brings together people, equipment, and facilities into a powerful system that is ready to respond to the emergency healthcare needs of the community. As a concept, the EMS system is refined continually.

This chapter examines the EMS system and describes the interactions of the systems' components. In addition, the chapter presents a prospectus of the prevailing challenges facing EMS systems.

▌ REVIEW QUESTIONS

Please circle one correct answer for each question.

1. Emergency Medical Services systems respond to the emergency healthcare needs of a community. Included in this complex process are: (C 1-1.1)

   a. people
   b. equipment
   c. facilities
   d. all of the above

2. A weak link in the EMS system continues to be provision for adequate funding. (C 1-1.7)

   a. true
   b. false

3. Compared to other industries, the attrition or turnover rate of prehospital personnel is: (C 1-1.5)

   a. equal
   b. higher
   c. lower
   d. not comparable

4. In EMS, most patient transportation is provided by: (C 1-1.1)

   a. air vehicles
   b. ground vehicles
   c. both of the above
   d. neither of the above

5. Emergency Medical Services systems must be evaluated continually to assure effectiveness. One method of evaluation is called: (C 1-1.5)

   a. quality insurance
   b. quality effectiveness
   c. quality assurance
   d. standardized inspection

6. An effective EMS system has numerous essential components. One of the most important components is: (C 1-1.6)

   a. system redesign
   b. medical direction
   c. protocols
   d. competitive salary range

7. To provide a quality, effective system of emergency medical care, which of the following must be in place? (C 1-1.7)

   a. laws
   b. regulations
   c. funding
   d. all of the above

8. Specific facility destination decisions should be based on: (C 1-1.1)

   a. the specific needs of the patient
   b. the capabilities of the various system facilities
   c. communication with medical control
   d. all of the above

9. It is proper for the EMT to always deliver the patient to the closest facility. (C 1-1.1)

   a. true
   b. false

10. The specialized group of professionals responsible for the development of criteria for identification of a trauma center is the: (C 1-1.7)

    a. American Medical Association
    b. American Society of Testing Materials
    c. Federal Communications Commission
    d. American College of Surgeons

11. Although not utilized in all areas of the country, the universal access number for emergency services is: (A 1-1.9)

    a. 411
    b. 119
    c. 991
    d. 911

12. Current methods for accessing the EMS system include all of the following **except**: (A 1-1.9)

    a. dialing a unique 7-digit telephone number
    b. standard 911 system
    c. enhanced 911
    d. dialing a universal 7-digit telephone number

13. Interhospital communication is an important component of the well-organized EMS system. (C 1-1.6)

    a. true
    b. false

14. Injury prevention programs ultimately lead to better utilization of EMS resources and improved patient outcome. (C 1-1.2)

    a. true
    b. false

15. A quality public information and education program can achieve: (C 1-1.2)

    a. a more efficient use of the EMS system
    b. reduction in accidental death and disability
    c. a reduction in the delay between onset of injury and start of emergency care
    d. all of the above

16. It is the physician's responsibility to be involved in all aspects of the patient care system. (C 1-1.6)

    a. true
    b. false

17. Specific areas of physician involvement include: (C 1-1.6)

    a. planning and protocols
    b. online medical direction and consultation
    c. audit and evaluation of patient care
    d. all of the above

18. The most common type of provider system is the: (C 1-1.2)

    a. Advanced Life Support System
    b. Basic Life Support System
    c. Advanced Cardiac Life Support System
    d. Pediatric Life Support System

19. The most common type of provider in the BLS system is the: (C 1-1.2)

    a. EMT-B
    b. EMT-Intermediate
    c. EMT-Paramedic
    d. first responder

20. Two nationally recognized levels of ALS providers are the: (C 1-1.2)

    a. first responder and EMT-Intermediate
    b. EMT-Intermediate and EMT-Paramedic
    c. EMT-BTLS Provider and EMT-BLS Provider
    d. EMT-Paramedic and Registered Physical Therapists

21. The EMS system model that involves layers of care is the: (C 1-1.1)

    a. dual response system
    b. tiered response system
    c. Advanced Support System
    d. definitive care system

22. One of the most critical challenges facing today's EMS systems is: (C 1-1.1)

    a. adequate funding
    b. inadequate number of consumers
    c. oversaturation of trained EMS professionals
    d. political perspectives

23. The modern EMS system has always had as its primary focus: (C 1-1.1)

    a. basic inhospital care
    b. prehospital emergency care
    c. advanced inhospital care
    d. nonemergency prehospital care

24. Private ambulance services may be: (C 1-1.1)

    a. nongovernmental
    b. nonhospital
    c. nonfire
    d. all of the above

Scenarios

Read each scenario. Write the answers to the corresponding questions in the space provided.

SCENARIO #1:

Your local EMS responds to the scene of a farm-related injury. Upon arrival at the scene, they find a 48-year-old male patient who is trapped underneath a tractor. The first ambulance on the scene is a volunteer basic service. When they arrive, they observe the local fire department volunteers setting up extrication equipment. The victim is freed from entrapment within three minutes of the arrival of the BLS unit. As the patient is being prepared for transport, a hospital-based ALS unit arrives on the scene. The patient is noted to have a change in consciousness and massive bleeding, and is turned over to the ALS unit for further treatment and transport.

1. What type of EMS-system model is demonstrated in this scenario?

   A tiered EMS model

2. Identify the EMS system components utilized to handle this scenario properly.

   volunteer basic EMS
   volunteer fire/Rescue
   Hospital based ALS ambulance

SCENARIO #2:

Your local dispatch center receives a call on a nonemergency line from a man who states that he is calling from a phone booth in the downtown area. He reports that he has just witnessed a robbery at the First Commerce Bank and that there were "shots fired." The dispatcher requests the caller's exact name, location, and the location of the incident. The first police unit on the scene announces that the scene is not secure and all rescue units should stage two blocks from the scene.

1. Which type of phone communication is NOT utilized in this scenario?

   911 was not used.

2. Which types of emergency providers will likely respond to this call?

   police, fire + EMS

CHAPTER 3 ANSWERS TO REVIEW QUESTIONS

1.	d	**6.**	b	**11.**	d	**16.**	a	**21.**	b
2.	a	**7.**	d	**12.**	d	**17.**	d	**22.**	a
3.	b	**8.**	d	**13.**	a	**18.**	b	**23.**	b
4.	b	**9.**	b	**14.**	a	**19.**	a	**24.**	d
5.	c	**10.**	d	**15.**	d	**20.**	b		

SCENARIOS SOLUTIONS

Scenario #1:

1. A tiered EMS model is represented in this scenario.

2. • Volunteer Basic EMS
   • Volunteer Fire/Rescue
   • Hospital Based ALS Ambulance

Scenario #2:

1. The 911 telephone communications was not used.
2. Police, Fire, and EMS units will respond to this call.

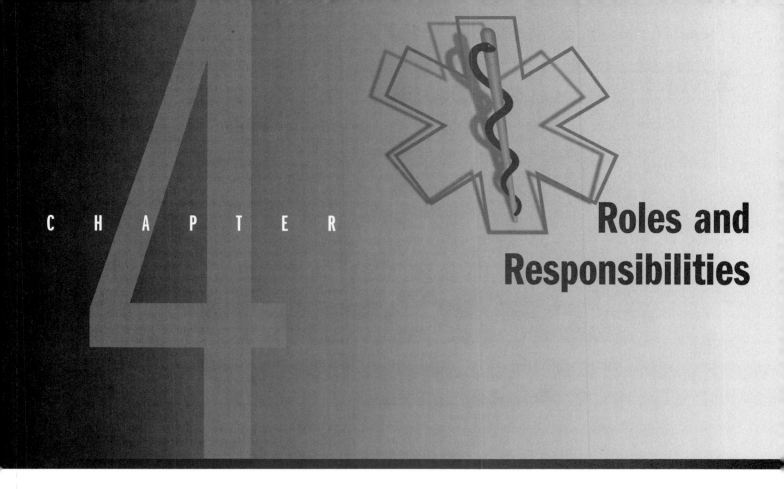

CHAPTER 4

Roles and Responsibilities

Reading Assignment: Chapter 4, pgs. 48–61

OBJECTIVES

1. Define the roles and responsibilities of the EMT-Basic (EMT-B) and differentiate these roles and responsibilities from those of other prehospital care providers.

2. Describe the roles and responsibilities of the EMT-B concerning personal safety and the safety of the crew, patients, and bystanders.

3. Describe various situations and settings that an EMT-B may encounter.

4. Describe the importance of personal attitude and conduct of the EMT-B.

5. Describe ethical dilemmas associated with EMS.

6. Describe the role of communication related to the EMT-B.

7. Discuss the role of the EMT-B as a healthcare professional.

8. Discuss the importance of teamwork and leadership for the EMT-B.

9. Differentiate between certification and licensure for the EMT-B.

10. Identify resources available to the EMT-B through professional organizations at the state and national levels.

INTRODUCTION

Emergency medical technicians must understand their roles and responsibilities in the EMS system. An integral portion of the EMT educational program enables the prospective EMT to make proper treatment and transport decisions. These decisions begin at the time the call is received and continue throughout delivery of the patient to the definitive healthcare center.

This chapter discusses the roles and responsibilities of the various levels of EMS responders. It also considers ethics, professionalism, teamwork, and professional organizations.

REVIEW QUESTIONS

Please circle one correct answer for each question.

1. An EMT is an individual who has been trained according to a national standard curriculum and who possesses the knowledge to provide initial assessment and emergency care for the ill and injured. (C 1-1.2)

    a. true
    b. false

2. The critical, first link in the chain of emergency care is the initiation of care by: (C 1-1.1)

    a. the emergency physician
    b. allied healthcare professionals
    c. informed and trained citizens
    d. critical incident debriefers

3. First responder training emphasizes: (C 1-1.1)

    a. initial assessment and basic emergency care
    b. shock management and bleeding control
    c. advanced airway management and oxygen administration
    d. traffic control at scene and personnel management

4. The EMT and all crew members must be prepared to perform their job skills at all times. Being prepared includes: (C 1-1.2)

    a. emotional and physical fitness
    b. having an excellent working knowledge of all equipment and its location on the emergency vehicle
    c. understanding the policies and procedures that define the EMS system
    d. all of the above

5. Emergency medical technicians must be knowledgeable of the geographic area, traffic patterns, and all traffic laws by which they must abide. (C 1-1.7)

    a. true
    b. false

6. Personal safety is the most important responsibility of the EMT.
    (C 1-1.3)

    a. true
    b. false

7. The systematic collection of information about the patient, both
    historical as well as that related to the current illness or injury, is
    known as: (A 3-2.20)

    a. observation
    b. intervention
    c. reassessment
    d. patient assessment

8. The EMT course teaches students to: (C 1-1.2)

    a. recognize life-threatening conditions
    b. evaluate the status of the patient
    c. provide appropriate treatment in a timely fashion
    d. all of the above

9. Prompt and effective treatment may include: (C 3-2.6)

    a. airway control
    b. control of bleeding, treatment of shock
    c. cardiopulmonary resuscitation
    d. all of the above

10. Safely and efficiently delivering the patient to the hospital is a
    component of treatment. The patient who is not treated en route to
    the hospital has a decreased chance of survival. (C 3-6.1)

    a. true
    b. false

11. An evaluation of the patient's illness or injury, as well as the
    location and availability of hospital resources, will assist in
    selecting: (C 1-1.1)

    a. the most appropriate medical facility
    b. the most appropriate attending physician
    c. the prospective rehabilitation center
    d. the need for completing a patient care report

12. The EMT must represent the patient and act in the patient's best
    interest until that responsibility can be passed on to another
    provider in the healthcare system. In doing so, the EMT is
    functioning as (a/an): (C 1-1.2)

    a. consultant
    b. advocate
    c. peer
    d. debriefer

13. The EMT's responsibilities include all the following except:
    (C 1-1.2)

    a. insuring that their uniform displays a professional image
    b. maintaining licensure in other medical professions
    c. demonstrating concern for personal safety
    d. maintaining good physical and emotional stability

14. Providing a verbal and or written report to the person who will be providing direct patient care is considered a: (C 1-1.5)

    a. third party release
    b. component of patient assessment
    c. continuum of care
    d. continuum of patient confidentiality

15. The EMT should be familiar with certain documents concerning ethics and confidentiality. They include: (A 1-1.8)

    a. the EMT Oath
    b. NAEMT Code of Ethics
    c. the Oath of Geneva
    d. all of the above

16. The EMT is responsible for knowing and complying with the laws and regulations that control prehospital care practice in: (C 1-1.7)

    a. his or her state(s) of employment
    b. the state(s) of his or her geographical region
    c. the county or parish in which he or she resides
    d. the collective states of the union

17. The process by which a governmental body grants permission to perform certain acts is known as: (C 1-1.7)

    a. licensure
    b. certification
    c. recertification
    d. continuing education

18. It is important for each EMT to understand the laws of their state primarily because: (C 1-1.7)

    a. he or she must continually update and renew their skills
    b. policies and procedures vary from state to state
    c. knowledge of the state laws will prevent litigation
    d. the EMT who is paid for his or her services will be protected by governmental immunity

19. The process by which an agency or association grants a document that attests to the accomplishment of a set of requirements is known as: (C 1-1.7)

    a. continuing education
    b. certification
    c. licensure
    d. reciprocity

20. Several national and state organizations are available for EMTs. The common goal of these organizations is to: (Chp. Obj. #10)

    a. promote professionalism within EMS services
    b. write national consensus EMS standards
    c. promote the professional status of the ER physician
    d. increase revenue for national nonprofit organizations

Scenarios

Read each scenario. Write the answers to the corresponding questions in the space provided.

SCENARIO #1:

Startled from sleep at 3 AM, you and the newest member of the crew leap from bed to answer a reported "severe nausea and vomiting" call. Since you know the area very well, you elect to drive to the scene. When you arrive at the scene, you immediately realize that the patient is seriously ill.

After an initial assessment, the decision is made to transport the patient to the definitive care facility in a timely manner. As the patient is placed into the ambulance, your partner asks directions to the hospital. You step out of the ambulance to assist your partner. When you return to the patient, you note that he has vomited and is no longer breathing. The EMS crew should conduct themselves in a professional manner.

1. Did both members of this crew act in a professional manner?

    _____

    _____

    _____

    _____

2. What actions of the crew members displayed a lack of professionalism?

    _____

    _____

    _____

    _____

SCENARIO #2:

You are called to the home of the town mayor. Dispatch informs you and your crew that this is a "domestic dispute" call. The local press—always at work—heard the call on the scanner and are waiting outside the home when you arrive on the scene. The police arrive simultaneously and they quickly secure the scene. As you transport the mayor to the ambulance, you are besieged with questions from the media.

1. What are your responsibilities to this patient, to yourself, and to the crew?

    _____

    _____

    _____

    _____

CHAPTER 4 ANSWERS TO REVIEW QUESTIONS

1. a	5. a	9. d	13. b	17. a
2. c	6. a	10. a	14. c	18. b
3. a	7. d	11. a	15. d	19. b
4. d	8. d	12. b	16. a	20. a

SCENARIOS SOLUTIONS

Scenario #1:

1. This scenario illustrates the importance of teamwork and coordination to a professional EMS crew. One critical performance area is driving the vehicle. To be a safe, effective, and professional emergency vehicle operator, the EMT must know how to operate the vehicle and find his or her way around the response area and to the major hospitals. In this case, the crew did not clarify, in advance of the call, which crew member was responsible for driving. One crew member drove to the scene and another, who didn't know how to find the hospital, was going to drive during the transport. These assignments and responsibilities should have been clearly identified before the call—not at the scene.

2. Once patient care has begun, a professional and effective EMS team maintains contact with the patient and monitors their status until they are delivered to the medical facility. In this case, the patient was left unattended at a critical time and may have actually died as a result of the inattention by this crew.

Scenario #2:

1. The EMT and crew responsibilities at this scene begin with personal safety. The police were present and secured the scene. Next the EMTs are responsible for appropriate and timely care of the patient, as well as for preserving patient confidentiality.

   Because of the political high profile of the patient involved, the EMTs must remain aware that patient care is the ultimate responsibility at this scene. The mayor's political affiliation should not, in any way, interfere with the rendering of quality patient care.

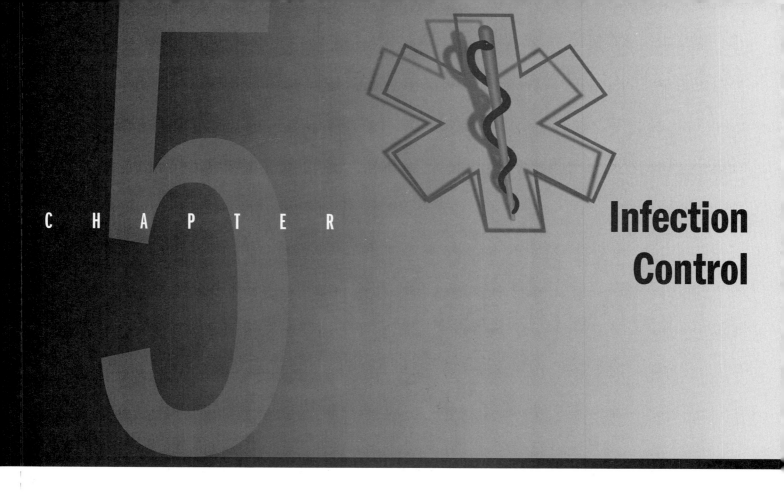

C H A P T E R

Infection Control

Reading Assignment: Chapter 5, pgs. 62–72

OBJECTIVES

1. Discuss the importance of body substance isolation (BSI).

2. Discuss common infectious diseases to which the EMT may be exposed.

3. Discuss the Occupational Safety and Health Administration (OSHA) precautions and Center for Disease Control and Prevention (CDC) guidelines for bloodborne pathogens.

4. Describe the steps that the EMT should take for personal protection from airborne and bloodborne pathogens.

INTRODUCTION

Healthcare providers, especially EMTs, are susceptible to bloodborne pathogen exposure because they often work in high-risk environments. This chapter discusses the need for EMTs to wear protective equipment while initiating patient care in situations where the chances of being exposed to pathogens are high such as cardiopulmonary resuscitation (CPR), intravenous (IV) insertion, trauma, and childbirth.

In addition, infectious diseases, modes of transmission, the OSHA standards, and employer responsibilities are addressed. The importance of body substance isolation is emphasized throughout the chapter.

REVIEW QUESTIONS

Please circle one correct answer for each question.

1. Situations where there is a high risk of exposure to pathogens include: (P 1-2.12)

   a. CPR and IV insertion
   b. trauma and childbirth
   c. open fractures and nosebleed
   d. all of the above situations pose risk of pathogen exposure

2. All of the following types of equipment can help protect the EMT from communicable disease exposure **except**: (C 1-2.7)

   a. gloves
   b. gowns
   c. lab coats
   d. masks

3. Communicable diseases are transmitted by all the following modes **except**: (C 1-2.7)

   a. direct contact and inhaling droplets
   b. contaminated needle puncture and bites
   c. blood transfusions and contaminated materials
   d. bronchial inhalers and new BSI devices

4. In the prehospital setting, the EMT may come into contact with patients who have a communicable disease. A communicable disease is one that can be passed or communicated from one organism to another. (C 1-2.7)

   a. true
   b. false

5. Which of the following common serious communicable diseases do not present a risk of exposure to the EMT? (C 1-2.8)

   a. meningitis
   b. tuberculosis
   c. hepatitis A or B
   d. measles

6. A term frequently used to describe communicable diseases is: (C 1-2.8)

   a. infectious diseases
   b. microorganisms
   c. immunizations
   d. exposure

7. Topics that must be included in OSHA-Required Bloodborne Pathogens Training Sessions include: (C 1-2.7)

   a. an overview of the modes of transmission of bloodborne pathogens
   b. principles regarding the control of risk and medical management of those who have been exposed
   c. appropriate cleaning techniques for equipment and appropriate packaging techniques for specimens
   d. all of the above are critical components of the OSHA-Required Bloodborne Pathogens Training Session

8. EMTs are especially susceptible to bloodborne pathogen exposure because they usually work in high risk environments. (C 1-2.7)

   a. true
   b. false

9. The federal organization responsible for publishing the regulations designed to protect employees who are at risk for exposure to bloodborne pathogens is: (C 1-2.7)

   a. Department of Human Resources
   b. OSHA
   c. CDC
   d. Federal Rural Health Association

10. Blood is not the only form of body fluid or substance that can contain microorganisms that may result in the transmission of communicable diseases. The simplest approach is to consider *any* substance from the body as being highly dangerous. Examples of body fluids include all the following **except**: (C 1-2.10)

   a. blood and urine
   b. feces and tears
   c. saliva and spinal fluid
   d. mucosa and bile

11. Bloodborne pathogens are microorganisms. Examples of bloodborne pathogens include: (C 1-2.10)

   a. viruses
   b. bacteria
   c. fungi
   d. all of the above

12. One communicable disease that is considered lifethreatening is: (C 1-2.8)

   a. measles
   b. AIDS
   c. chickenpox
   d. herpes simplex

13. Communicable diseases are transmitted through a variety of ways. These include: (C 1-2.7)

    a. direct contact such as through a handshake, kissing, or sexual intercourse
    b. inhaling droplets such as when the EMT inhales the infected moisture that the patient exhales or coughs out
    c. contaminated needle puncture such as when a healthcare professional administers an injection to a patient
    d. a, b, and c are correct

14. Infection is caused by organisms called: (C 1-2.8)

    a. pathogens
    b. antibiotics
    c. toxins
    d. antigens

15. Most diseases are contagious for only a portion of the time. This contagious time is called the: (C 1-2.7)

    a. communicable period
    b. pathogen protection
    c. exposure time
    d. incubation period

16. In addition to the OSHA mandated "Exposure Control Plan," the employer must also provide training for its personnel as soon as they are retained and at least: (C 1-2.7)

    a. monthly
    b. weekly
    c. annually
    d. twice yearly

17. In addition to the employer requirements, the EMT has important responsibilities to ensure a safe working environment. These responsibilities include: (C 1-1.3)

    a. removal of gloves and jewelry and washing hands thoroughly for at least 30 seconds after each patient contact
    b. wiping down the vehicle floor, walls, and stretcher at least once a day with a 1:10 mixture of household bleach and water or an appropriate commercial cleaning solution
    c. wiping down frequently used items such as radios, stethoscopes, monitors, and oxygen tanks
    d. all of the above are EMT responsibilities

18. To clean properly after blood spillage, absorb the spill with disposable paper towels or linens and clean the area with: (C 1-2.9)

    a. a mixture of 100% bleach and water
    b. a 1:10 mixture of bleach and water
    c. 100% sterile water
    d. hot, soapy water

19. The pneumatic antishock garment (PASG) should be cleaned according to manufacturer's recommendations that usually include: (C 1-2.13)

    a. scrubbing the garment with 100% sterile water
    b. scrubbing the garment with hot, soapy water
    c. scrubbing the garment with warm, soapy water, thorough rinsing and drying time
    d. scrubbing the garment with 100% ethyl alcohol

20. Body substance isolation is a process used by healthcare providers to separate or isolate themselves from potentially dangerous body substances. This is most effectively accomplished through: (C 1-2.8)

    a. immunizations
    b. handwashing
    c. using bacteriocidal lotion
    d. wearing prescription eyeglasses

21. Disposable gloves: (C 1-2.8)

    a. should be used by all EMS personnel prior to initiating emergency care
    b. are especially appropriate when the EMT may come into contact with body fluids, especially blood or bloody body fluids
    c. should fit tightly at the wrist
    d. all of the above

22. If a patient is known or suspected to have tuberculosis: (C 1-2.7)

    a. a high efficiency particulate air (HEPA) respirator should be worn by the EMT
    b. transport the patient in an internally ventilated ambulance
    c. the EMT should wear a surgical mask
    d. the EMT should not consider having the patient wear an HEPA respirator

23. Resuscitation equipment (pocket masks, bag-valve masks, and other ventilation devices) should be immediately available to all EMS personnel to minimize the need for: (C 1-2.7)

    a. CPR
    b. mouth-to-mouth resuscitation
    c. disposable items
    d. disinfecting equipment

24. Use of protective devices on a regular basis will ensure that the risk of exposure to a communicable disease is minimized. (C 1-2.9)

    a. true
    b. false

25. Before starting work in the prehospital setting, EMTs should make sure that they are up to date on all of the recommended immunizations. These include all of the following **except**: (C 1-2.9)

    a. HAB (*Haemophilus influenzae*-B)
    b. DPT (diphtheria-pertussis-tetanus)
    c. a tetanus booster every 10 years
    d. MMR (measles, mumps, and rubella)

Scenario

Read each scenario. Write the answers to the corresponding questions in the space provided.

SCENARIO #1:

Your EMT crew receives a call to a domestic dispute. Upon arrival at the scene, you find a twenty-five-year old male who has sustained numerous knife wounds, two of which are spurting bright red blood. The bystanders report that he has been notified within the past week that he is human immunodeficiency virus (HIV) positive. He is conscious and slightly combative. The EMT notes that the patient is perspiring profusely and that there are needle tracks on his arms.

1. This situation contains caution flags for the EMT. What are they?

_____

_____

_____

_____

2. What steps should the EMT take to protect themselves and others from the danger in this situation?

_____

_____

_____

_____

3. Discuss the proper management and patient care for this patient.

_____

_____

_____

_____

_____

CHAPTER 5 ANSWERS TO REVIEW QUESTIONS

1. d	**6.** a	**11.** d	**16.** c	**21.** d
2. c	**7.** d	**12.** b	**17.** d	**22.** a
3. d	**8.** a	**13.** d	**18.** b	**23.** b
4. a	**9.** b	**14.** a	**19.** c	**24.** a
5. d	**10.** d	**15.** a	**20.** b	**25.** a

SCENARIO SOLUTIONS

Scenario #1:

1. The EMT should exercise extreme personal safety precautions due to the nature of the call and because the patient is combative. The patient may have been exposed to HIV from sharing needles and to possibly hepatitis C from blood transfusions.

2.3. The EMT crew should observe strict BSI precautions while properly managing this patient. These issues are not mutually exclusive. The following actions should be taken:

1) Have the scene secured before entering and ensure that the patient is treated in a professional manner.

2) Explain to the patient that the precautions are medically necessary.

3) Provide appropriate emergency care including management of airway, breathing, and circulation.

4) Avoid direct contact with any of the patient's bodily fluids.

5) Wear gloves and gowns.

6) Wear eye protection.

7) Wear a dust or surgical mask.

8) Calmly reassure the patient during treatment and transport.

9) Open the windows in the ambulance to facilitate airflow and ventilation in the patient compartment.

10) Thoroughly disinfect the inside of the ambulance, any equipment used in treating the patient, and the cot and dispose of bed linen appropriately.

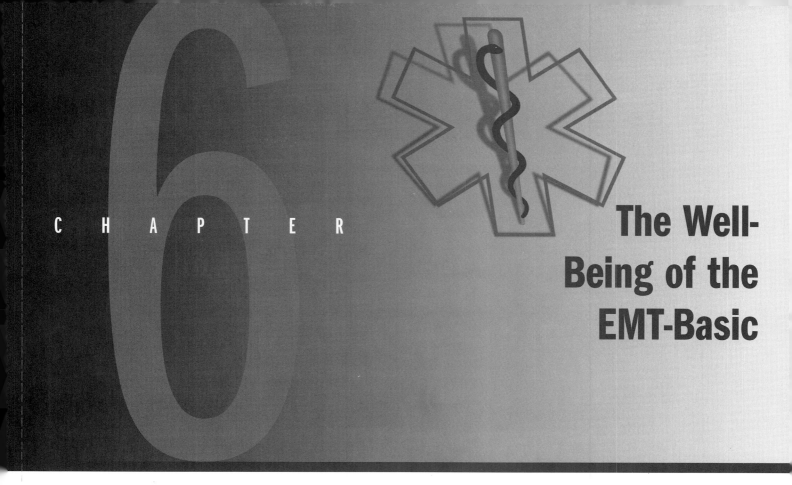

CHAPTER 6

The Well-Being of the EMT-Basic

Reading Assignment: Chapter 6, pgs. 74–98

OBJECTIVES

1. Explain the importance of surveying the scene.

2. Discuss the importance of body substance isolation (BSI).

3. List personal protective equipment and considerations necessary for special situations including:

   - Hazardous Materials
   - Rescue Operations
   - Exposure to Bloodborne Pathogens
   - Violent Scenes
   - Exposure to Airborne Pathogens
   - Crime Scenes

4. Discuss the possible reactions that a patient and their family may exhibit when confronted with death and dying.

5. State the steps that the EMT-Basic will take to approach a family confronted with death and dying.

6. List the possible reactions that the EMT-Basic may experience when faced with trauma, illness, death, and dying.

7. State the possible reactions that the family of the EMT-Basic may exhibit due to their indirect involvement with EMS.

8. Recognize the signs and symptoms of critical incidence stress debriefing.

9. List the steps that the EMT-Basic should take to prevent, reduce, and alleviate stress.

INTRODUCTION

Emergency Medical Services is one of the most challenging and fulfilling healthcare professions. Emergency medical technicians begin their careers filled with new knowledge, skills, and opportunities and are typically excited, challenged, and eager to discover all that the EMS professions have to offer.

The fast-paced, action-oriented world of EMS is filled with various stressors that inevitably impact the neophyte and the veteran EMT. It is critical for the EMT to be cognizant of the stresses of EMS so that his or her coping mechanisms can be called upon to recognize the signs of stress.

The EMT must choose to be safety conscious, to take precautions, and to maintain a balanced, healthy lifestyle. The express purpose of this chapter is to teach the EMT how to take care of himself or herself.

REVIEW QUESTIONS

Please circle one correct answer for each question.

1. The first action of an EMT arriving on the scene is to: (C 1-2.7)

    a. survey the scene
    b. initiate the patient care report
    c. contact Medical Control
    d. direct traffic

2. All of the following steps are part of the scene survey **except**: (C 1-2.7)

    a. assess the scene for hazards
    b. note the number of patients
    c. note the mechanism of injury
    d. decide if the patient's family requires notification

3. Continued scene security can be assured by which of the following? (C 1-2.7)

    a. reassess ambulance or rescue vehicle location
    b. look for hazards around the patient location
    c. use of specialized equipment such as turnout gear or breathing apparatus
    d. all of the above

4. You arrive on the scene of a one vehicle accident. The female driver is restrained and still in the vehicle. You notice a diaper bag and baby bottle lying in the floor of the vehicle. Your next action would be to: (C 3-1.5)

    a. call for more ambulances immediately
    b. notify medical direction or dispatch to initiate disaster protocols
    c. direct your partner to search for the infant
    d. check for a passenger list

5. Emergency Medical Technicians learn how to predict injuries best by noting the: (C 3-1.4)

    a. mechanism of injury
    b. vehicle damage detail
    c. type of vehicles involved
    d. type(s) of weapons involved

6. Additional extrication or rescue considerations may be required when dealing with the entrapment of a patient. These considerations include all of the following **except**: (C 3-1.1)

   a. is specialized equipment needed
   b. does a specialized rescue team need to be called
   c. thorough scene survey is extremely important
   d. hysterical patients pose no threat to scene control

7. After assuring that the scene is safe, the EMT's primary responsibility is: (C 3-1.3)

   a. initiation of patient care reports
   b. providing medical care to the patient
   c. to request rescue teams for extensive or heavy rescue
   d. coordinate patient care with police officers

8. Violent scenes should always be controlled by law enforcement personnel before the EMT provides patient care because: (C 1-2.9)

   a. most EMTs are not prepared to intervene in violent situations
   b. it is the EMT's responsibility to provide law enforcement
   c. patient care is not rendered if the perpetrator of the crime is still on the scene
   d. the EMT is not trained to recognize dangerous situations

9. On occasion, EMTs may be called to a scene that turns out to be criminal in nature. Whether or not patient care is delivered, the EMTs have an additional responsibility to preserve the crime scene and act as witnesses. (C 1-2.10)

   a. true
   b. false

10. The EMT should take the same path in and out of a suspected crime scene to: (C 1-2.10)

    a. enhance patient care
    b. avoid disturbing evidence
    c. stay out of the police officers' way
    d. maintain orientation at an unfamiliar scene

11. A mental defense mechanism that creates a buffer between the reality of the person's present condition and the reality of their actually dying from that condition is known as: (C 1-2.1)

    a. regression
    b. conversion reaction
    c. denial
    d. manic depression

12. "Why Me?" expresses the emotion known as:

    a. anger
    b. conversion reaction
    c. denial
    d. manic depression

13. When facing a catastrophic illness or injury, some patients react initially by the process known as "bargaining." The person may: (C 1-2.1)

    a. bargain with God
    b. bargain with their family
    c. bargain with the medical professionals
    d. all of the above

14. Family and close friends at the scene may also respond in a wide range of actions and emotions. (C 1-2.2)

    a. true
    b. false

15. Family members should be allowed to stay with the patient in the patient compartment on the way to the hospital in the ambulance. (C 1-2.2)

    a. true
    b. false

16. Hearing is the first sense to be lost. (C 1-2.3)

    a. true
    b. false

17. If a family member arrives at the scene before the patient dies: (C 1-2.2)

    a. do not arrange for them to see the patient
    b. arrange for them to see the patient
    c. do not give them any information about the patient
    d. do not allow the family to talk to the patient

18. Some family members may want to touch or hold the body after death. Do not deny this request unless: (C 1-2.2)

    a. it is a crime scene or it compromises your care or local protocol
    b. the family member appears too upset to deal with the situation
    c. the medical examiner or coroner arrives on the scene
    d. the family member appears mature enough to deal with the situation

19. When EMTs are responding to an emergency or faced with a stressful scene, information is relayed to the brain through their _____ senses. (C 1-2.5)

    a. two
    b. four
    c. five
    d. six

20. Physiologic reaction simply means that the normally functioning human body will respond in a physical way. (C 1-2.5)

    a. true
    b. false

21. In stressful situations, epinephrine (adrenaline) and other chemicals are released to prepare the body to deal with the situation. Physiologic responses may include all of the following **except**: (C 1-2.1)

   a. respirations and blood pressure increase
   b. muscles tighten, pupils dilate
   c. glucose is released into the blood for immediate energy
   d. heart rate decreases

22. The type of response described in the questions 19-21 is often referred to as: (C 1-2.1)

   a. "feed or breed"
   b. "fight or flight"
   c. hyperactivity
   d. abnormal and unhealthy

23. Acute stress results from a single event or activity while chronic stress results from short-term exposure to one or more sources of stress. (C 1-2.1)

   a. true
   b. false

24. While responding to an emergency or on the scene, an EMT may experience signs and symptoms of the normal response to a stressful situation. These include: (C 1-2.1)

   a. upset stomach and dry mouth
   b. nausea and vomiting
   c. shivering or shakes and sweating
   d. all of the above

25. Some EMTs suppress their emotions and refuse to talk about them or participate in debriefing following a critical incident or traumatic event. This type of unhealthy suppression of emotions and thoughts may lead to: (C 1-2.5)

   a. Post-traumatic Stress Disorder (PTSD)
   b. Chronic Disorder Counseling (CDC)
   c. Pre-traumatic Stress Denial (PTSD)
   d. Post-trial Strain Disorder (PTSD)

26. In recent years, a process known as Critical Incident Stress Management (CISM) has been introduced to EMS with great success. (C 1-2.5)

   a. true
   b. false

27. It is possible to prevent, reduce, and alleviate stress that leads to distress. Managing your stress level is one area of your profession that is 100% your responsibility. All of the following suggestions will assist in stress management **except**: (C 1-2.4)

   a. balancing your life with work, recreation, family, friends
   b. recognizing that your personality includes physical, mental, emotional, and spiritual needs
   c. maintaining a positive attitude at all times
   d. working out your frustrations by excessive alcohol intake

Scenario

Read each scenario. Write the answers to the corresponding questions in the space provided.

SCENARIO #1:

Your EMT- B crew is dispatched to a domestic violence call. Upon arrival at a local bar, a man meets you at the door to the bar and states, "Hurry! A man has been shot and is bleeding to death!" You and your partner run into the bar to assess the situation at the scene. The patient is lying on the floor surrounded by a pool of blood. As you approach the patient, you see a man standing in the corner holding a gun.

Suddenly, you hear him yell, "If you touch him, I will kill you!" You see that the man standing in the corner is pointing a handgun at you.

1. How could this situation have been avoided?

   _____

   _____

   _____

   _____

2. How can you undertake the resolution of this situation?

   _____

   _____

   _____

   _____

CHAPTER 6 ANSWERS TO REVIEW QUESTIONS

1. a	7. b	13. d	19. c	25. a
2. d	8. a	14. a	20. a	26. a
3. d	9. a	15. b	21. d	27. d
4. c	10. b	16. b	22. b	
5. a	11. c	17. b	23. b	
6. d	12. a	18. a	24. d	

SCENARIO SOLUTIONS

Scenario #1:

1. Your involvement in this dangerous situation could have been averted if you had remembered the guidelines for managing violent scenes. Those guidelines are as follows:
   • Violent scenes should always be controlled by law enforcement personnel before the EMT provides patient care.
   • EMTs are not trained, equipped, or paid to intercede in violent situations, nor is it the EMT's responsibility to provide law enforcement.

- One must be especially cautious if the perpetrator of the crime is still on the scene.
- Be observant for potential weapons.
- Be alert to bystander or family reactions.

If the EMTs had kept these guidelines in mind, the initial reactions in this scenario would have been safer. Other prudent measures would include:

- Turn off the lights and siren as you near the scene.
- Stop at least a block away from the address and verify the presence of law enforcement officers.
- If the police have not arrived, you should notify dispatch of your arrival on scene and advise that you are waiting in the ambulance for the police to arrive. As you wait, be very alert for signs of activity in or around the scene.
- Only if the police have arrived should you proceed to park at the scene.
- Identify yourselves as "EMS personnel." People who are upset may mistake EMS personnel for law enforcement officers.

2. To attempt to resolve this scenario, you should indicate that you will leave immediately. Ask the man to put the gun down so that you and your partner can leave. Since the injured man is obviously in need of immediate care, ask if you can take the patient with you to the hospital. Abide by the answer you receive and leave immediately.

Return to the ambulance and drive away without lights or sirens, rendering appropriate care to the patient, if he was allowed to leave the scene with you. You then radio dispatch and medical control immediately and provide an update of the both the scene situation and the patient status. In addition, you now realize the importance of personal and scene safety!

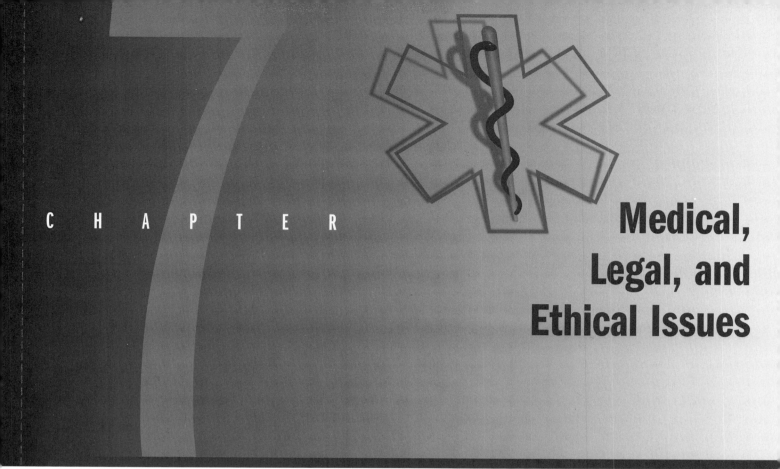

Medical, Legal, and Ethical Issues

C H A P T E R

Reading Assignment: Chapter 7, pgs. 99–111

OBJECTIVES

1. Define the EMT's scope of practice.

2. Discuss the importance of Do Not Resuscitate (DNR) orders or advanced directives including state or local provisions regarding application by EMS personnel.

3. Define consent and discuss methods of obtaining consent.

4. Differentiate between expressed and implied consent.

5. Explain the role of consent of minors in providing emergency care.

6. Discuss the implications for the EMT when a patient refuses transportation.

7. Discuss the issues of abandonment, negligence, and assault and battery, and their implications to the EMT.

8. State the conditions necessary for the EMT to have a duty to act.

9. Explain the importance, necessity, and legality of patient confidentiality.

10. Discuss the considerations of the EMT in issues of organ retrieval.

11. Differentiate the actions that an EMT should take to assist in the preservation of a crime scene.

12. State the conditions that require an EMT to notify local law enforcement officials.

INTRODUCTION

The decision to become a part of the EMS system can be a rewarding one. As with most professions, along with rewards come risks. One of the less positive aspects of the EMS profession is the risk of litigation.

The EMT can minimize the risk of being sued by gaining an understanding of the U.S. legal system, the EMT's scope of practice, the rights of the patient, and the importance of delivering appropriate care. This chapter presents pertinent aspects of medical and legal considerations for the prehospital care provider.

REVIEW QUESTIONS

Please circle one correct answer for each question.

1. One of the negative aspects to the pursuit of a career in EMS is: (C 1-3.1)

   a. the risk of being sued
   b. the EMT's scope of practice
   c. the rights of the patient
   d. the importance of delivering appropriate care

2. The U.S. legal system is very complex compared to other countries. (C 1-3.1)

   a. true
   b. false

3. There are two basic types of law: criminal and civil (or tort). Criminal law deals with: (C 1-3.1)

   a. issues that are not criminal in nature, including breach of contract, divorce, and torts
   b. crime and punishment wherein the government sues an individual who is accused of committing the crime
   c. individuals and/or companies who sue each other
   d. statutes (federal) enacted by Congress

4. In most states, specific legislation that defines the scope of practice of the Basic EMT is known as: (C 1-3.1)

   a. the State Medical Control Act
   b. the EMT Act of 1968
   c. the Good Samaritan Act
   d. the State EMS Law

5. The EMT has legal responsibilities to the: (C 1-3.1)

   a. patient
   b. medical director
   c. public
   d. all of the above

6. The EMT is responsible to the medical director for any treatment that is either provided or omitted in the prehospital care setting. (C 1-3.1)

   a. true
   b. false

7. Because EMTs cannot be certain how the legal system will view the actions they have taken, all EMTs should strongly consider purchasing their own: (C 1-1.2)

   a. interactive EMS computer software
   b. intubation equipment
   c. malpractice insurance
   d. private health and dental insurance

8. Liberties that every person can reasonably expect to be guaranteed by the legal system in the US are called: (C 1-3.2)

   a. rights
   b. advanced decisions
   c. entitlements
   d. prohibitions

9. Local law may require that patients be given the opportunity to establish a mechanism for refusal of resuscitation efforts through a "living will." Collectively, these decisions are known as: (C 1-3.2)

   a. physician issuances
   b. entitlements
   c. advanced directives
   d. citizen statements

10. Laws and protocols governing DNR orders vary from state to state. (C 1-3.2)

   a. true
   b. false

11. In general, DNR orders are issued at the request of the: (C 1-3.2)

   a. patient
   b. patient's surrogate decision maker
   c. either a or b
   d. only a is true

12. To withhold resuscitation efforts: (C 1-3.2)

   a. a written statement from the patient's spouse is required
   b. a written DNR order from a physician is required
   c. a written DNR order from a nurse practitioner is required
   d. a written DNR order from a clergy member is required

13. Providing emergency care when the patient does not consent to the treatment can result in charges against the EMT for: (C 1-3.3 and 1-3.7)

   a. assault
   b. battery
   c. liability for abuse
   d. all of the above

14. If the EMT touches a person without their consent, even if the EMT justifiably believes that the action is necessary to save the patient's life, he or she may be charged with: (C 1-3.3 and 1-3.7)

   a. battery
   b. libel
   c. slander
   d. assault

15. To refuse care, the patient must be: (C 1-3.6)

   a. of legal age
   b. mentally competent
   c. conscious
   d. all of the above

16. If a patient refuses care, the EMT should: (C 1-3.6)

   a. leave the scene immediately, without comment
   b. forcibly restrain and transport the patient
   c. calmly inform the patient of the possible consequences of refusing treatment
   d. always utilize the doctrine of "implied consent"

17. If the patient continues to refuse care, the EMT should: (C 1-3.6)

   a. inform medical command, as directed by local protocol
   b. should carefully explain to the patient the possible diagnosis
   c. should carefully explain to the patient the treatment that is indicated, and the possible consequences if he or she is not treated
   d. all of the above

18. If all of these efforts fail and the patient still refuses care, the EMT should: (C 1-3.6)

   a. accept the patient's decision and document the event
   b. inform the patient that the decision is no longer his
   c. threaten the patient with arrest for criminal mischief
   d. all the above

19. The authority to restrain and transport patients against their will generally rests only with: (C 1-3.4)

   a. a probate judge
   b. a police officer
   c. a spouse and/or significant other
   d. the EMS system Medical Director

20. Permission to treat minor children, even against the child's wishes, is usually under the jurisdiction of the: (C 1-3.5)

   a. child
   b. parents or legal guardian
   c. county sheriff
   d. family attorney

21. Expressed consent means that: (C 1-3.4)

    a. a patient can voluntarily express consent to be treated only if they are at least 18 years of age
    b. the patient must be informed via written documentation of the procedures and treatments to be administered
    c. if the patient is unconscious, the EMT should specifically ask for this consent
    d. the consent must be informed

22. In which of the following situations would implied consent be applicable? (C 1-3.4)

    a. a patient who is unconscious and is bleeding profusely
    b. a patient who is describing his accident to bystanders
    c. a patient who nods in the affirmative when asked if he or she needs medical help
    d. a 14-year-old pregnant patient exhibiting extreme anxiety

23. Emancipated minors include those minors who are: (C 1-3.5)

    a. over the age of 16 years
    b. freed from parental control
    c. maintained and supported by only one of the parents
    d. pregnant

24. Abandonment: (C 1-3.7)

    a. is failure to continue to care for the patient, once it has been initiated
    b. abandonment can result in the EMT being subject to liability for negligence
    c. abandonment can take many forms
    d. all of the above

25. All of the following statements are examples of abandonment **except**: (C 1-3.7)

    a. the EMT initiates care and leaves the patient, or turns him or her over to someone who has less training
    b. the patient is left unattended for a brief period of time and his or her condition worsens or additional injury is sustained
    c. the EMT fails to transfer information to the receiving facility regarding the patient's history, treatment, or current condition
    d. the EMT responds to and completes an ambulance call in an appropriate and efficient manner

26. The EMT is expected to provide the same level of care as any other competent EMT with equivalent training. Failure to provide this standard of care is defined as: (C 1-3.7)

    a. abandonment
    b. negligence
    c. claim
    d. duty to act

27. A duty to act: (C 1-3.8)

    a. implies a contractual or legal obligation to provide patient care
    b. may be formal, such as an ambulance service contracting to provide emergency care to the citizens of the community
    c. can be implied, such as an EMT initiating treatment of the patient
    d. all of the above

28. A breach of the duty to act can be shown by all of the following **except**: (C 1-3.8)

    a. offering evidence that the EMT did not conform to the standard of care by rendering inappropriate care

    b. offering evidence that the EMT failed to act at all

    c. offering evidence that the EMT acted beyond the scope of practice

    d. offering evidence that the EMT acted as a reasonably prudent EMT would in the same or similar circumstances

29. Patient confidentiality is a critical component of prehospital emergency care. The following statement is true regarding patient confidentiality: (C 1-3.9)

    a. The patient has no right to expect information regarding the ambulance call to be kept confidential.

    b. Confidential information may include any history elicited through interview of the patient or their family.

    c. Assessment findings and treatment rendered are not examples of confidential patient information.

    d. Medical information regarding a minor requires no release form be signed.

30. The EMT's responsibility in organ donation is to: (C 1-3.10)

    a. identify the patient as an potential donor

    b. establish communication with medical command and relay this information

    c. provide appropriate care to maintain organ viability

    d. all of the above

31. The EMT's responsibilities at a crime scene include all of the following **except**: (C 1-3.11)

    a. providing emergency care of the patient as a last priority

    b. avoid disturbing any item at the scene unless patient care requires it

    c. observing and documenting anything unusual at the scene

    d. avoid cutting through holes in clothing that may be the result of gunshot wounds or stabbings

32. Each state has its own legislation mandating that certain conditions be reported to the appropriate authorities. It is essential that the EMT be aware of these reporting requirements. Common reporting requirements include all of the following **except**: (C 1-3.12)

    a. abuse of children and the elderly

    b. victims of domestic violence

    c. crimes such as sexual assault

    d. overdose by drug addicts

33. Methods of providing medical direction that permit the EMT to practice include: (C 1-3.1)

    a. Online—through telephone and radio communications

    b. Offline—through standing orders or protocols

    c. Both a and b are true

    d. Neither a nor b is true

34. What action should the EMT take if an unsigned written "DNR" order is presented at the scene of a cardiac arrest? (A 1-3.13)

   a. Leave the scene immediately.
   b. Initiate resuscitation efforts.
   c. Initiate only rescue breathing.
   d. Have the family member sign the document in your presence.

35. Two elements that must be proven in a successful negligence suit include: (C 1-3.7)

   a. a duty to act; a breach of the duty to act occurred
   b. a duty to act; no breach of the duty occurred
   c. the patient experienced no injury; proximate cause
   d. the EMT breached the duty to act; no injury occurred

Scenarios

Read each scenario. Write the answers to the corresponding questions in the space provided.

SCENARIO #1:
You and your partner respond, in a BLS ambulance, to the scene of a motor vehicle accident. En route to the scene, your vehicle proceeds through an intersection against the red light at a speed of 50 mph. At the center of the intersection, your vehicle collides with a car that had not cleared the intersection. Both your partner and the driver of the other vehicle are injured.

1. What is your required standard of care when operating this ambulance?

2. What steps could you take to protect yourselves from legal risks?

SCENARIO #2:
You and your BLS ambulance crew are responding to the scene of a "possible cardiac arrest." En route to the call, you and your partner witness a two-car accident involving six victims.

1. What action is legally correct regarding your situation?

continued

2. What are the legal problems that could be encountered should you elect to stop at the scene of the motor vehicle accident (MVA)?

_____

_____

_____

_____

CHAPTER 7 ANSWERS TO REVIEW QUESTIONS

1.	a	**8.**	a	**15.**	d	**22.**	a	**29.**	b
2.	a	**9.**	c	**16.**	c	**23.**	b	**30.**	d
3.	b	**10.**	a	**17.**	d	**24.**	d	**31.**	a
4.	d	**11.**	c	**18.**	a	**25.**	d	**32.**	d
5.	d	**12.**	b	**19.**	b	**26.**	b	**33.**	c
6.	a	**13.**	d	**20.**	b	**27.**	d	**34.**	b
7.	c	**14.**	a	**21.**	d	**28.**	d	**35.**	a

SCENARIOS SOLUTIONS

Scenario #1:

1. The required standard is to drive with due regard for the safety of others, and to avoid unsafe driving practices.

2. You should avoid breach of duty by maintaining the standard of care in all cases of patient supervision. You should realize that you have a duty to protect not only the patient, but also your co-workers and bystanders.

Scenario #2:

1. The appropriate action in this situation is for you to continue on to the scene of your original call. You should immediately contact your dispatch center to report the MVA, as well as to state your observations of the scene.

2. If you elect to stop at the scene of the MVA, you have abandoned the patient who originally called for help.

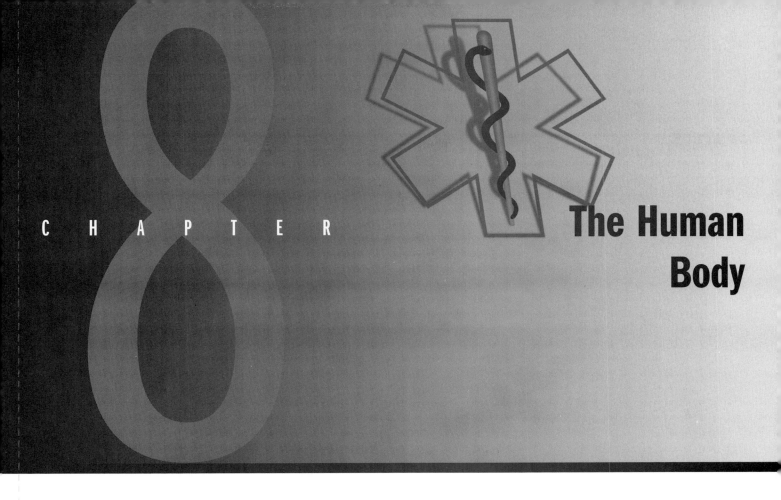

CHAPTER 8

The Human Body

Reading Assignment: Chapter 8, pgs. 112–136

OBJECTIVES

1. Describe the various components of medical terminology, including medical abbreviations.

2. Identify the following directional terms: medial, lateral, proximal, distal, superior, inferior, anterior, posterior, midline, right and left, apices, midclavicular, bilateral, midaxillary.

3. Describe the structure and function of the following major body systems: respiratory, circulatory, musculoskeletal, integumentary, nervous, and endocrine.

INTRODUCTION

Prehospital care focuses on "assessment-based" patient care interventions. The foundation of patient assessment is a working knowledge of the anatomy (structure) and physiology (function) of the human body. Patient assessment and appropriate use of proper medical terminology are critical components of EMS education for the prehospital healthcare provider.

This chapter reviews anatomical terms and the skeletal and body systems, and introduces the EMT-B to medical terms. This information enables the EMT-B to begin building the foundation for quality patient assessment and intervention.

REVIEW QUESTIONS

Please circle one correct answer for each question.

1. The language unique to the medical profession is known as: (C 1-4.1)

   a. medical jargon
   b. medical terminology
   c. medical lingo
   d. communication

2. The root word "append" means: (C 1-4.1)

   a. appendix
   b. surgical
   c. prescript
   d. postscript

3. A prefix is made up of one or more syllables and is located: (C 1-4.1)

   a. at the beginning of the word
   b. at the end of the word
   c. in the middle of the word
   d. none of the above is true

4. A suffix is located: (C 1-4.1)

   a. at the beginning of the word.
   b. at the end of the word
   c. in the middle of the word
   d. none of the above

5. Terms used to describe directional anatomy are based upon the assumption that the body is in the anatomical position. In this position: (C 1-4.1)

   a. the patient stands upright and faces forward
   b. the arms are down at the sides
   c. the palms face forward
   d. all of the above are correct

6. When the terms right and left are used: (C 1-4.1)

   a. they refer to the patient's right and left
   b. they refer to the EMT's right and left
   c. they refer to the EMT's left and right
   d. they refer to the patient's upper extremities

7. The term torso refers to the: (C 1-4.1)

   a. trunk of the body
   b. chest
   c. midline
   d. head

8. The heart is medial to the: (C 1-4.1)

    a. pelvis
    b. right arm
    c. femur
    d. mouth

9. The elbow is: (C 1-4.1)

    a. distal to the wrist
    b. lateral to the shoulder
    c. proximal to the wrist
    d. proximal to the shoulder

10. The heart is superior to the: (C 1-4.1)

    a. shoulders
    b. cervical spine
    c. pelvis
    d. mouth

11. The heart is inferior to the: (C 1-4.1)

    a. knees
    b. skull
    c. pelvis
    d. diaphragm

12. The mid-axillary line is an imaginary line running: (C 1-4.1)

    a. horizontally through the shoulders
    b. vertically from the middle of the armpit to the ankle
    c. from the chest to the back
    d. from the nose to the pelvis

13. The abdomen is located: (C 1-4.1)

    a. anterior to the spine
    b. posterior to the heart
    c. inferior to the pelvis
    d. lateral to the chest

14. Clavicles are:

    a. superior to the heart
    b. posterior to the liver
    c. inferior to the pelvis
    d. lateral to the chest

15. The term used to refer to both sides is: (C 1-4.1)

    a. unilateral
    b. quadrilateral
    c. bilateral
    d. trilateral

16. The term meaning towards the back is: (C 1-4.1)

    a. ventral
    b. superior
    c. bactral
    d. dorsal

17. Plantar refers to the: (C 1-4.1)

    a. palm of the hand
    b. sole of the foot
    c. dorsal side of the foot
    d. medial side of the wrist

18. Prone refers to: (C 1-4.1)

    a. lying face up
    b. lying face down
    c. sitting up
    d. lateral recumbent

19. Supine refers to: (C 1-4.1)

    a. lying face up
    b. lying face down
    c. sitting up
    d. lateral recumbent

20. The patient was placed in the Fowler's position on the stretcher. This indicates that the patient was: (C 1-4.1)

    a. lying face up
    b. lying face down
    c. sitting up
    d. lateral recumbent

21. The musculoskeletal system: (C 1-4.2)

    a. is the framework for the body
    b. protects vital internal organs
    c. provides for body movement
    d. all of the above

22. The two major components of the musculoskeletal system are: (C 1-4.2)

    a. bones and cartilages
    b. skeleton and muscles
    c. joints and muscles
    d. heart and lungs

23. The skeleton is made up of: (C 1-4.2)

    a. 233 bones
    b. 189 bones
    c. 206 bones
    d. 256 bones

24. The skeleton is divided into: (C 1-4.2)

    a. seven components
    b. eleven components
    c. eight components
    d. five components

25. Joints are the points at which: (C 1-4.2)

    a. tendons connect to other tendons
    b. ligaments connect to other ligaments
    c. bones connect to other bones
    d. cartilage connects to bone

26. There are two major types of joints. They include the ball and socket joint and the: (C 1-4.2)

    a. hinged joint
    b. shoulder joint
    c. false joints
    d. diastasis

27. The four areas of the skull are the frontal, occipital, temporal, and parietal, and are located respectively: (C 1-4.2)

    a. anterior, posterior, sides, and top
    b. posterior, sides, anterior, and top
    c. posterior, anterior, sides, and top
    d. anterior, sides, posterior, and top

28. The lower jaw is the only moveable face bone. The medical term for the lower jaw is: (C 1-4.2)

    a. the zygomatic arch
    b. the maxilla
    c. the mandible
    d. the orbit

29. The five vertebral areas of the spinal (vertebral) column are the cervical, the thoracic, the lumbar, the sacral, and the coccygeal, respectively. Collectively, the column is composed of 33 bones. The correct number of vertebrae per section is: (C 1-4.2)

    a. 7, 12, 5, 5, and 4
    b. 5, 12, 7, 5, and 4
    c. 7, 12, 4, 5, and 5
    d. 5, 12, 7, 5, and 4

30. The major organs and blood vessels contained within the thorax are the: (C 1-4.2)

    a. heart, lungs, diaphragm, aorta, and the superior and inferior vena cavae
    b. heart, lungs, kidneys, aorta, and the superior and inferior vena cavae
    c. heart, lungs, kidneys, aorta, and the superior and inferior aorta
    d. heart, lungs, cerebellum, aorta, and the superior and inferior vena cavae

31. Each upper extremity consists of the: (C 1-4.2)

    a. shoulder and arm
    b. elbow and forearm
    c. wrist and hand
    d. all of the above

32. The pelvis rests at the inferior section of the torso and is made up of the: (C 1-4.2)

    a. iliac crest
    b. ischium
    c. pubic symphysis
    d. all of the above

33. The bone of the thigh is called the: (C 1-4.2)

    a. tibia
    b. fibula
    c. femur
    d. patella

34. Voluntary muscles are also referred to as: (C 1-4.2)

    a. unconscious muscles
    b. smooth muscles
    c. myocardial muscles
    d. skeletal muscles

35. Involuntary muscles are also referred to as: (C 1-4.2)

    a. instinctive muscles
    b. smooth muscles
    c. myocardial muscles
    d. skeletal muscles

36. Cardiac muscle is unique because it can: (C 1-4.2)

    a. be controlled voluntarily
    b. generate its own contractions
    c. tolerate interruption of the blood supply
    d. regenerate after cell and tissue damage

37. The respiratory system performs the critical function of supplying the body with oxygen and eliminating carbon dioxide. (C 1-4.2)

    a. true
    b. false

38. The respiratory system is divided into the upper and lower airways. Air enters the upper airway through the ____ and _____ and then passes into the _____. (C 1-4.2)

    a. nose, mouth, pharynx
    b. mouth, pharynx, nose
    c. epiglottis, nose, larynx
    d. nose, mouth, larynx

39. The vocal cords, which produce sound, are contained within the _____. (C 1-4.2)

    a. air passages
    b. larynx
    c. trachea
    d. thyroid cartilage

40. Assessing a patient's breathing requires a determination of respiratory: (C 1-4.2)

    a. rate and rhythm
    b. quality
    c. depth (tidal volume)
    d. all of the above

41. The major components of the cardiovascular system are: (C 1-4.2)

    a. heart, blood, blood vessels
    b. heart, lungs
    c. aorta, pleura, vena cavae
    d. heart, lungs, veins

42. The heart is made up of three layers: the epicardium (outer layer), the myocardium (middle layer), and the endocardium (inner layer). The _____ is the muscle that contracts. (C 1-4.2)

    a. endocardium
    b. pericardium
    c. myocardium
    d. epicardium

43. The heart is supplied with oxygenated blood by the: (C 1-4.2)

    a. coronary arteries
    b. superior vena cavae
    c. inferior vena cavae
    d. descending aorta

44. The carotid arteries originate from the aorta to supply the _____ with blood. (C 1-4.2)

    a. lower extremities
    b. heart
    c. thigh
    d. head

45. The major artery of the upper arm is the _____ artery. (C 1-4.2)

    a. medial
    b. radial
    c. posterior tibial
    d. brachial

46. Two major veins of the body are the _____ _____, which deliver oxygen-poor blood from the body into the right atrium. (C 1-4.2)

    a. vena cavae
    b. capillary veins
    c. pulmonary circulation
    d. pulmonary artery

47. The exchange of carbon dioxide waste products and oxygen in the lungs occurs between the _____ and the capillaries. (C 1-4.2)

    a. alveoli
    b. pleura
    c. endocardium
    d. carina

48. _____ blood cells make up the largest component of the cell content in blood and are responsible for carrying oxygen from the lungs to the tissues and carbon dioxide from the tissues to the lungs. (C 1-4.2)

    a. hemoglobin
    b. white
    c. red
    d. platelet

49. The _____ system is the control center of the body, evaluating internal and external stimuli and directing body functions in response to these stimuli. (C 1-4.2)

    a. integumentary
    b. nervous
    c. cardiovascular
    d. endocrine

50. Involuntary functions, such as respiration, circulation, and digestion, are carried out by the _____ nervous system. (C 1-4.2)

    a. endocrine
    b. autonomic
    c. cardiovascular
    d. integumentary

51. The skin, also referred to as the _____ system, is the largest organ of the body. (C 1-4.2)

    a. integumentary
    b. nervous
    c. cardiovascular
    d. endocrine

52. The skin is made up of three layers: the epidermis, dermis, and subcutaneous layer. The _____ is the outermost layer of skin. (C 1-4.2)

    a. dermis
    b. epidermis
    c. fascia
    d. adipose

53. The endocrine system secretes chemicals called _____. (C 1-4.2)

    a. endorphins
    b. hormones
    c. endocrines
    d. glands

54. The circulatory system delivers hormones to the target tissues, where they: (C 1-4.2)

    a. regulate growth and produce energy
    b. maintain fluid balance and respond to stress
    c. manage reproductive functions
    d. all of the above

55. Two major hormones are: (C 1-4.2)

    a. adrenalin and insulin
    b. epinephrine and hemoglobin
    c. insulin and heparin
    d. glucose and insulin

56. The abdominal cavity is divided into ____ sections. (C 1-4.2)

    a. three
    b. four
    c. two
    d. six

57. The abdominal cavity is lined by a thin membrane called the _____. (C 1-4.2)

    a. mesentery
    b. peritoneum
    c. endocardium
    d. perineum

58. The kidneys lie behind the abdominal cavity in what is referred to as the: (C 1-4.2)

  a. retroperitoneal space
  b. peritoneum superior
  c. umbilicus ligamentous
  d. mesenteric arteriosus

59. The term bilateral means: (C 1-4.1)

  a. pertaining to both sides
  b. only one side
  c. four extremities
  d. lower extremities

60. The xiphoid process is the: (C 1-4.1)

  a. inferior tip of the sternum
  b. posterior tip of the sternum
  c. superior tip of the sternum
  d. proximal tip of the sternum

Scenario

Read each scenario. Write the answers to the corresponding questions in the space provided.

SCENARIO #1:

Your EMT crew is called to a residence where a painter has fallen from a scaffold. He was painting the trim on the second floor dormer windows when he lost his footing and fell to the ground. Your patient is not conscious when you arrive. You note a large laceration on the back of the patient's head. He is lying on his back on the ground.

After assessing the patient further, you find that he also has a swollen, deformed area near the elbow on the left forearm that is not bleeding profusely, a large cut on the inside of his right upper leg that is bleeding heavily, and his lower right leg is deformed.

1. Which major body systems may be involved as a result of these injuries?

_____

_____

_____

_____

2. Describe the location of the laceration on the patient's head.

_____

_____

_____

_____

continued

3. In what position was the patient found?

_____

_____

_____

_____

4. Describe the location of the forearm injury.

_____

_____

_____

_____

CHAPTER 8 ANSWERS TO REVIEW QUESTIONS

1.	b	**13.**	a	**25.**	c	**37.**	a	**49.**	b
2.	a	**14.**	a	**26.**	a	**38.**	a	**50.**	b
3.	a	**15.**	c	**27.**	a	**39.**	b	**51.**	a
4.	b	**16.**	d	**28.**	c	**40.**	d	**52.**	b
5.	d	**17.**	b	**29.**	a	**41.**	a	**53.**	b
6.	a	**18.**	b	**30.**	a	**42.**	c	**54.**	d
7.	a	**19.**	a	**31.**	d	**43.**	a	**55.**	a
8.	b	**20.**	c	**32.**	d	**44.**	d	**56.**	b
9.	c	**21.**	d	**33.**	c	**45.**	d	**57.**	b
10.	c	**22.**	b	**34.**	d	**46.**	a	**58.**	a
11.	b	**23.**	c	**35.**	b	**47.**	a	**59.**	a
12.	b	**24.**	a	**36.**	b	**48.**	c	**60.**	a

SCENARIO SOLUTIONS

Scenario #1:

1. The nervous system, cardiovascular system, integumentary system, musculoskeletal system, and the respiratory system may be involved.
2. The laceration on the back of the patient's head is found in the occipital region of the skull.
3. The patient was found in the supine position.
4. The forearm injury is located distal to the elbow or could be stated as a proximal forearm injury.

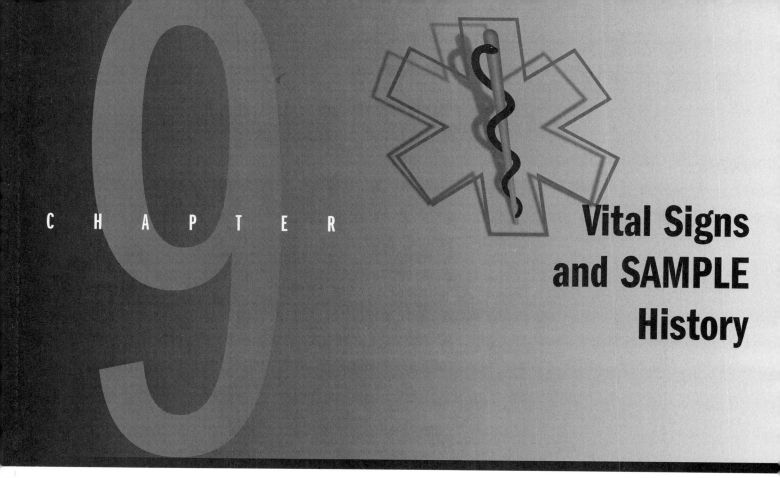

CHAPTER 9

Vital Signs and SAMPLE History

Reading Assignment: Chapter 9, pgs. 137–150

OBJECTIVES

1. Identify components of vital signs and distinguish differences from symptoms.

2. Describe methods of obtaining a pulse and identify the information that can be gathered in the assessment.

3. Describe methods of obtaining an evaluation of respirations and identify the information gathered in the assessment.

4. Describe method of assessing blood pressure and define systolic and diastolic.

5. Identify the equipment used to assess blood pressure.

6. Describe the difference between auscultation and palpation.

7. Describe the assessment of skin color and temperature.

8. Describe the assessment of level of consciousness using the AVPU method.

9. Describe pupil reaction and differentiate between constriction and dilation.

10. Describe the method used to obtain a SAMPLE history and describe the importance of the information gathered.

INTRODUCTION

Accurate and early assessment of vital signs and medical history are critical components of an EMS call. This chapter equips the EMT student with the information needed to obtain these components in an efficient and professional manner.

Although life-threatening problems must be managed initially, vital signs and patient history may govern patient care for the course of the call. Therefore, this chapter describes a working knowledge of vital sign assessment and patient history collection will be described in this chapter.

REVIEW QUESTIONS

Please circle one correct answer for each question.

1. Signs are things that can be seen, heard, smelled, measured or felt concerning a patient's illness or injury. Examples of signs are: (C 1-5.24)

    a. hemorrhaging
    b. pain
    c. nausea
    d. weakness

2. Symptoms are things that have to be related by the patient. An example of a symptom is: (C 1-5.24)

    a. noise as the patient breathes
    b. chest pain
    c. deformity
    d. external bleeding

3. Vital signs generally include all of the following **except**: (C 1-5.1)

    a. respirations, pulse
    b. blood pressure, temperature
    c. level of consciousness, pulse
    d. pupil reaction, weight

4. The wave of blood flowing through the vessels of the body as the heart beats is called the: (C 1-5.6)

    a. blood pressure
    b. pulse
    c. capillary refill
    d. AVPU

5. The pulse can be felt wherever a(n) _____ lies close to the skin and can be pressed against any underlying firm tissue, such as bone or cartilage. (C 1-5.5)

    a. vein
    b. artery
    c. capillary
    d. aorta

6. Pulses are most often assessed in the _____ artery in the wrist at the base of the thumb or in the _____ artery on either side of the front of the neck. (C 1-5.5)

    a. carotid, brachial
    b. carotid, femoral
    c. radial, carotid
    d. femoral, carotid

7. Pulses are evaluated for: (C 1-5.6)

    a. rate
    b. character
    c. rhythm
    d. all of the above

8. Pulse rate is the number of beats per minute and may vary among individuals. The normal pulse rate for an adult at rest is: (C 1-5.6)

    a. 60–100 beats per minute
    b. 80–100 beats per minute
    c. 100–120 beats per minute
    d. 130–140 beats per minute

9. A rapid pulse is called tachycardia. If an adult's pulse rate falls below 60 beats per minute, the rate is called: (C 1-5.5)

    a. bradycardia
    b. tachycardia
    c. dysrhythmia
    d. arrhythmia

10. A strong pulse is considered a "full" pulse and an extremely strong pulse is described as: (C 1-5.7)

    a. feeble
    b. bounding
    c. regular
    d. thready

11. When the pulse wave feels weak and feeble, the pulse is said to be: (C 1-5.7)

    a. irregular
    b. bounding
    c. regular
    d. thready

12. Pulse rhythm refers to the intervals between the beats of the heart. If the beats are not constant, the pulse is: (C 1-5.7)

    a. inconsistent
    b. irregular
    c. thready
    d. regular

13. When assessing the patient's pulse, if the pulse is irregular or the patient is a child, always count for: (P 1-5.33)

    a. one full minute
    b. thirty seconds
    c. two minutes
    d. ninety seconds

14. When assessing the femoral pulse, a greater amount of pressure may have to be exerted than at the carotid and radial pulses because the femoral artery lies deeper below the skin surface than at other pulse sites. (P 1-5.33)

    a. true
    b. false

15. The process of expelling the air in the lungs is called: (C 1-5.2)

    a. inhalation
    b. exhalation
    c. expiration
    d. both b or c is true

16. The respiratory rate is the number of respirations in one minute. The normal respiratory rate for an adult is between: (C 1-5.3)

    a. 30 and 60 breaths per minute
    b. 12 and 24 breaths per minute
    c. 4 and 40 breaths per minute
    d. 16 and 32 breaths per minute

17. Respiratory _____ refers to the amount of air that is exchanged with each breath. (C 1-5.3)

    a. quality
    b. quantity
    c. rate
    d. regularity

18. To assess respiratory character, watch the movement of the chest and listen to the patient breathe. If the patient has to exert effort to take each breath, the respirations are described as: (P 1-5.32)

    a. shallow
    b. labored
    c. regular
    d. stridorous

19. The pressure exerted on the walls of the arteries as blood is forced through the circulatory system by the contraction of the heart is called the: (C 1-5.20)

    a. pulse pressure
    b. diastolic pressure
    c. systolic pressure
    d. ventricular pressure

20. The difference between the systolic and diastolic pressure is the: (C 1-5.20 and 21)

    a. pulse pressure
    b. blood pressure
    c. systolic pressure
    d. diastolic pressure

21. Two pieces of equipment are used to assess the blood pressure. One is the stethoscope and the other piece of equipment is the: (C 1-5.19)

    a. sphygmomanometer
    b. pulse oximeter
    c. automatic monitor
    d. glucometer

22. Under normal conditions, the most accurate method for assessing blood pressure is: (P 1-5.36 and C 1-5.22)

    a. percussion
    b. auscultation
    c. palpation
    d. automatic monitor

23. Skin color can be a good indicator of: (C 1-5.10)

    a. heart function
    b. lung function
    c. cerebral function
    d. a and b

24. Pale skin may indicate: (C 1-5.10)

    a. shock
    b. heart attack
    c. emotional distress
    d. all of the above

25. Cyanosis may indicate poor oxygen levels in the blood and may be described as a: (C 1-5.9 and 10)

    a. bluish discoloration of the skin
    b. yellowish discoloration of the skin
    c. reddish discoloration of the skin
    d. greenish discoloration of the skin

26. A red skin color may be caused by: (C 1-5.9 and 10)

    a. high blood pressure
    b. low-grade fever
    c. extensive blood loss
    d. liver disease

27. Skin temperature is assessed by touching the patient's skin with the: (C 1-5.8 and 5.34)

    a. side of the assessor's hand
    b. back of the assessor's hand
    c. front of the assessor's hand
    d. front of the patient's hand

28. Normal skin is generally: (C 1-5.11)

    a. warm and dry
    b. very hot and dry
    c. cool and moist
    d. hot and moist

29. A patient with unusually cool skin may be experiencing: (C 1-5.12)

    a. shock
    b. heat exhaustion
    c. exposure to cold
    d. all of the above

30. The AVPU system is used to describe the patient's level of consciousness. (C 3-2.2)

    a. true
    b. false

31. If the patient is aware of the time, the place where he or she is located, and the current date, and can recognize persons around him or her, then the patient is said to be: (C 3-2.2)

   a. alarmed
   b. attentive
   c. animated
   d. oriented

32. Under normal circumstances, and with few exceptions, the pupils of both eyes will appear equal in size. (C 1-5.16)

   a. true
   b. false

33. All of the following statements are true regarding pupil reaction with the **exception** of: (C 1-5.18)

   a. The speed in which the constriction or dilation takes place should be the same.
   b. Pupils that react differently may indicate injury and may be slow to react or not react at all.
   c. A person assessing pupil reaction should note if the patient has a prosthetic device (glass eye) or if the patient is blind.
   d. Unequal pupil size is always an abnormal finding.

34. It is important that the EMT obtain a medical history regarding the patient. If the patient is unconscious or otherwise unable to provide the information, the information should be obtained from: (A 1-5.31)

   a. law enforcement officers who are present at the scene
   b. neighbors or co-workers who are present at the scene
   c. relatives who are present at the scene or who live with the patient
   d. the patient's clergy, if present at the scene

35. When using the acronym "S A M P L E" in obtaining the patient's medical history, the EMT will understand that the "S" in the acronym signifies: (C 1-5.23)

   a. signs and symptoms
   b. vital signs
   c. allergies
   d. significant past events

36. When using the acronym "S A M P L E" in obtaining the patient's medical history, the EMT will understand that the "A" in the acronym signifies: (C 1-5.23)

   a. signs and symptoms
   b. vital signs
   c. allergies
   d. significant past events

37. When using the acronym "S A M P L E" in obtaining the patient's medical history, the EMT will understand that the "M" in the acronym signifies: (C 1-5.23)

   a. signs and symptoms
   b. medications
   c. allergies
   d. significant past events

38. When using the acronym "S A M P L E" in obtaining the patient's medical history, the EMT will understand that the "L" in the acronym signifies: (C 1-5.23)

   a. signs and symptoms
   b. medications
   c. allergies
   d. last meal

39. Which of the following locations is usually NOT used to take the pulse of an adult? (C 1-5.5)

   a. femoral artery
   b. brachial artery
   c. carotid artery
   d. radial artery

40. Normally, the patient's pupils will _____ when exposed to bright light. (P 1-5.35 and C 1-5.15 and 17)

   a. dilate
   b. constrict
   c. become unequal
   d. not react

Scenario

Read each scenario. Write the answers to the corresponding questions in the space provided.

SCENARIO #1:

A patient is complaining of a severe headache. He awoke at 3 AM with severe discomfort "between his eyes." The patient is alert and oriented and his face appears red. The patient's respiratory rate is 16 and not distressed.

When assessing the patient's pulse, you note that it is very strong and seems to have a long pause between some beats. The pulse rate, when evaluated for a minute, is 120.

When you are checking the patient's blood pressure, you pump the cuff up to 200 mm Hg and can still hear the pulse. After inflating the cuff to 240 mm Hg, you determine the blood pressure is 220/130.

1. Did you find anything to indicate respiratory compromise?

   _____

   _____

   _____

   _____

2. Is the patient's pulse regular?

   _____

   _____

   _____

   _____

continued

3. Is the patient's pulse rate within normal range?

_____

_____

_____

4. Is the patient's blood pressure within normal range?

_____

_____

5. How will the patient's vital signs guide you in the assessment of this patient?

_____

_____

_____

_____

CHAPTER 9 ANSWERS TO REVIEW QUESTIONS

1. a	9. a	17. b	25. a	33. d
2. b	10. b	18. b	26. a	34. c
3. d	11. d	19. c	27. b	35. a
4. b	12. b	20. a	28. a	36. c
5. b	13. a	21. a	29. d	37. b
6. c	14. a	22. b	30. a	38. d
7. d	15. d	23. d	31. d	39. b
8. a	16. b	24. d	32. a	40. b

SCENARIO SOLUTIONS

Scenario #1:

1. There were no indications of respiratory compromise in this patient.
2. The patient's pulse is irregular.
3. The patient's pulse rate was not within normal range (normal pulse rate for the adult patient is 60–100)
4. The patient's blood pressure is elevated.
5. Vital signs are valuable in assessing the patient's status. The blood pressure gives an indication of the efficiency of the heart. Evaluation of the pulse intervals determines whether the heart has a regular rhythm. The rate determines if the heart beats within the normal range. Evaluation of the respirations determines if the patient needs immediate airway assistance. The SAMPLE history aids in determining if there is a history of similar problems or diagnosed disease, such as hypertension.

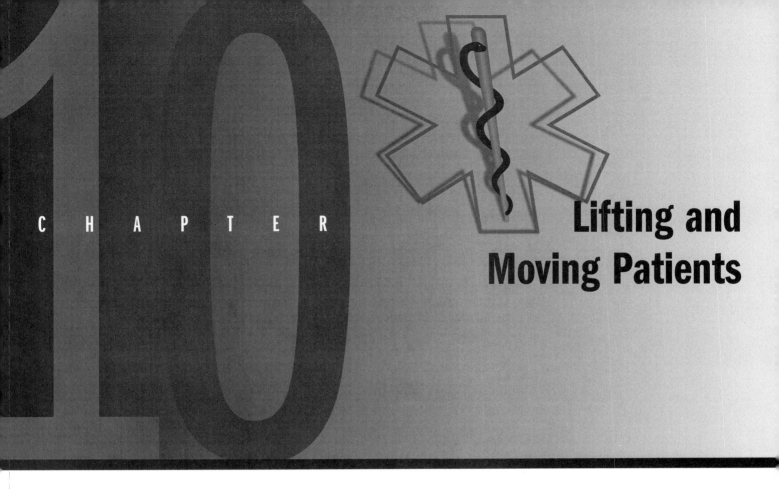

Lifting and Moving Patients

Reading Assignment: Chapter 10, pgs. 151–176

OBJECTIVES

1. Define body mechanics.

2. Discuss guidelines and safety precautions that must be followed when lifting a patient.

3. Describe guidelines and safety precautions for carrying patients and equipment.

4. Describe the safe lifting of cots and stretchers.

5. Describe correct and safe carrying procedures on stairs.

6. State the guidelines for reaching, pushing, and pulling and their applications.

7. Identify seven standard patient carrying devices and their applications.

8. State three situations that require the use of an emergency move.

INTRODUCTION

Frequently, many EMT-Bs are injured in the process of lifting and moving patients because they attempt to lift or move a patient improperly. A variety of patient conditions, as well as environmental considerations, factor into the decision for patient "packaging." The specific piece of equipment and the appropriate lift-and-carry method should be selected after considering all of the factors.

The design of this chapter is to establish guidelines that will help the EMT to minimize the possibility of sustaining an injury due to lifting and moving patients.

REVIEW QUESTIONS

Please circle one correct answer for each question.

1. The human body is capable of lifting tremendous amounts of weight. EMTs regularly lift patients weighing as much as 300 pounds. (C 1-6.1)

   a. true
   b. false

2. The long bones are the strongest in the body. Of these bones the largest is the: (C 1-6.2)

   a. scapula
   b. femur
   c. humerus
   d. pelvis

3. The best stance for lifting a stretcher is: (C 1-6.3 and P 1-6.14)

   a. always get as far as possible from the stretcher
   b. keep your arms and the weight you are lifting 20 inches from your body
   c. stand with your feet about shoulder's width apart and place one foot slightly in front of the other
   d. bend at the knees while keeping your feet close together and side by side

4. When lifting, use the back, not the legs. (C 1-6.2)

   a. true
   b. false

5. Twisting or swinging motions are the safest and most efficient techniques to use when lifting patients. (C 1-6.4)

   a. true
   b. false

6. _____ injuries due to improper lifting techniques are among the most common causes of injury and disability for prehospital personnel. (C 1-6.4)

   a. head
   b. back
   c. knee
   d. neck

7. Use a minimum of ___ people to lift, even if a one rescuer stretcher is being used. (C 1-6.3)

   a. one
   b. two
   c. four
   d. three

8. When carrying equipment by hand, try to balance the weight and bulk evenly from side to side. When carrying only one piece of equipment, resist the tendency to lean to the ___ to compensate for the imbalance. (C 1-6.5)

   a. front
   b. side
   c. back
   d. medial

9. One of the most difficult carries an EMT must perform is to carry a patient ___ up a stairway. (C 1-6.6)

   a. frontwards
   b. sideways
   c. backwards
   d. forwards

10. To minimize the possibility of injuries while reaching, the EMT should: (C 1-6.7)

   a. over extend
   b. keep the back straight
   c. twist
   d. stretch

11. Use your ___ muscles when log-rolling the patient. (C 1-6.8)

   a. hamstring
   b. shoulder
   c. gluteal
   d. triceps

12. When pulling a patient, the EMT should keep the line of pull through the ___ of his or her body by bending the ___. (C 1-6.9)

   a. center, knees
   b. center, arms
   c. medial, back
   d. periphery, ankles

13. Guidelines for pushing or pulling patients include: (C 1-6.9)

   a. pushing whenever possible, rather than pulling
   b. pulling whenever possible, rather than pushing
   c. lifting whenever possible, rather than pulling
   d. pushing and pulling from an overhead position

14. All moves fall into one of three categories. These categories include all of the following **except**: (C 1-6.10)

   a. emergency
   b. urgent
   c. nonurgent
   d. convalescent

15. A patient should be moved promptly by an emergency move only when there is an immediate danger to the patient or the rescuers, including: (C 1-6.11)

    a. fire or danger of fire
    b. danger of explosives or other hazardous materials
    c. inability to protect the patient from other hazards at the scene
    d. all of the above

16. If the patient is on the floor or ground, an in-line drag can be used to pull the person to safety. The most common in-line drags include the: (C 1-6.11)

    a. clothing drag
    b. sheet drag
    c. blanket drag
    d. all of the above

17. The motor vehicle collision is an example of a scene that frequently requires a(n) _____ move or "rapid extrication." (C 1-6.10)

    a. emergent
    b. urgent
    c. nonemergent
    d. convalescent

18. The majority of moves required for patients are of a nonurgent nature. (C 1-6.10)

    a. true
    b. false

19. The piece of equipment used most often for moving patients is the: (C 1-6.12)

    a. wheeled stretcher
    b. stairchair
    c. Stokes basket
    d. scoop stretcher

20. Stair chairs are designed for patients who can assume a sitting position while being carried from a residence or scene to the ambulance. Stair chairs must not be used for patients who are: (P 1-6.14 and A 1-6.13)

    a. unconscious
    b. alert
    c. medical rather than trauma patients
    d. suspected of having a fractured arm

21. Which piece of equipment would be used to lift and transport a multiple trauma patient? (A 1-6.13)

    a. flexible stretcher
    b. stair chair
    c. long backboard
    d. scoop stretcher

22. The backboard's uses include: (A 1-6.13)

    a. spinal immobilization
    b. moving patients
    c. removing the patient from a vehicle during rapid extrication
    d. all of the above

23. The patient with a suspected spinal injury who is moved with a scoop stretcher should immediately be placed on a long backboard for immobilization. (C 1-6.13)

   a. true
   b. false

24. Unresponsive patients without suspected spine injury should be placed in the recovery position, which is: (C 1-6.12)

   a. on their back
   b. on their left side
   c. in a prone position
   d. in a seated position

25. A patient with chest pain, chest discomfort, or difficulty breathing should never be walked to the ambulance. (C 1-6.13)

   a. true
   b. false

Scenarios

Read each scenario. Write the answers to the corresponding questions in the space provided.

SCENARIO #1:

An elderly female is found supine in the basement complaining of hip pain. The patient stated the pain started as she made a bad step from the bottom stair. She states she did not fall but sat down and then lay on the floor. She is alert and oriented. She states she has had similar problems before.

1. What device(s) would be appropriate to move the patient from the basement?

_____

_____

_____

_____

2. What device would be the most comfortable for the patient? Why?

_____

_____

_____

_____

SCENARIO #2

You and your EMT crew witness a MVA while returning to the station to await the next call. You note that there is one patient involved in the accident and you elect to care for the patient. You note that the patient is A&O X4 and has sustained an open fracture of the right femur. Your partner informs you that there is gasoline spilling under the car.

continued

1. What type move will be best used in this scenario?

   _____

   _____

   _____

   _____

2. Explain your answer to question #1.

   _____

   _____

   _____

   _____

CHAPTER 10 ANSWERS TO REVIEW QUESTIONS

1.	a	**6.**	b	**11.**	b	**16.**	d	**21.**	c
2.	b	**7.**	b	**12.**	a	**17.**	b	**22.**	d
3.	c	**8.**	b	**13.**	a	**18.**	a	**23.**	a
4.	b	**9.**	c	**14.**	d	**19.**	a	**24.**	b
5.	b	**10.**	b	**15.**	d	**20.**	a	**25.**	a

SCENARIOS SOLUTIONS

Scenario #1:

1. The appropriate device(s) would be the long backboard and/or scoop stretcher.
2. The scoop stretcher would probably be more comfortable due to its ease of application and the limited movement of the patient.

Scenario #2:

1. The emergency move.
2. The emergency move is the proper move to use in this scenario because of the danger presented by this scene to you, your partners, and the patient.

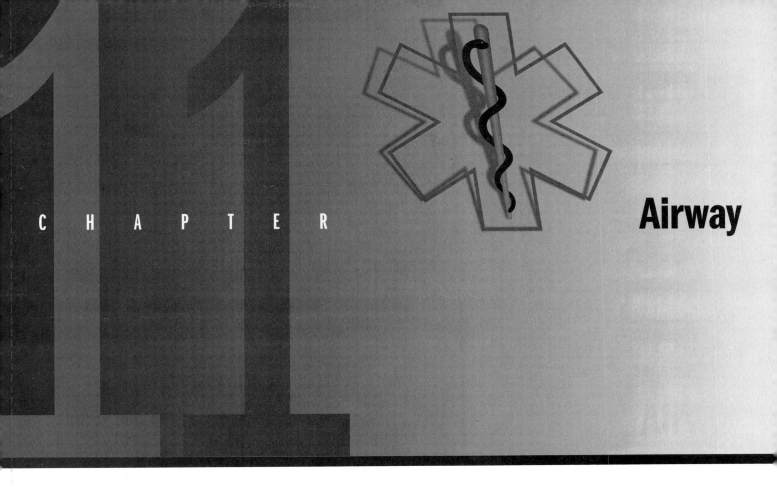

CHAPTER 11

Airway

Reading Assignment: Chapter 11, pgs. 177–200

OBJECTIVES

1. Identify major respiratory structures and relate these structures to the function of the respiratory system.

2. Explain why artificial ventilation and airway management skills take priority over most of the other basic life-support skills.

3. Assess whether a patient is breathing adequately, and appropriately manage a patient who needs ventilatory assistance.

4. Explain the rationale for giving a high-inspired oxygen concentration to patients who need it—even if there is a possibility of depression of ventilatory drive.

5. Identify indications for and demonstrate the proper use of common airway equipment, including the pocket mask, bag-valve-mask (BVM) device, nasopharyngeal and oropharyngeal airway, and flow-restricted, oxygen-powered ventilator device.

6. Describe and demonstrate techniques for opening and protecting the airway, including the head-tilt–chin-lift, jaw thrust, and Sellick maneuvers.

7. Describe the importance of suctioning equipment and demonstrate proper suctioning technique.

■ INTRODUCTION

Airway management and ventilation are among the most important skills an EMT must master. Proper assessment of airway compromise and rapid interventions have a dramatic impact on patient outcome. Airway and ventilation assessments take place on every call.

Airway management techniques change rapidly. Endotracheal intubation is now an optional skill for the EMT-B. Performance of this skill requires special training and practice as well as frequent retraining.

This chapter begins with an overview of the anatomy, physiology, and pathophysiology of the respiratory system. It also discusses airway and ventilatory assessments, equipment and skills needed for airway management and artificial ventilation, and common problems the EMT must manage in the field.

■ REVIEW QUESTIONS

Please circle one correct answer for each question.

1. The lowest (most inferior) part of the pharynx is called the: (C 2-1.1)

   a. hypopharynx
   b. lungs
   c. oropharynx
   d. nasopharynx

2. The most common cause of an obstructed airway in an unconscious patient is the: (C 2-1.5)

   a. saliva
   b. mucus
   c. tongue
   d. teeth

3. A leaf-shaped structure located just above the larynx that prevents food and liquids from entering the trachea (windpipe) during swallowing is called the: (C 2-1.1)

   a. epiglottis
   b. oropharynx
   c. carina
   d. tongue

4. At the level of the sternal angle, the trachea divides into left and right mainstem bronchi. This division is called the: (C 2-1.1)

   a. carina
   b. larynx
   c. voice box
   d. thyroid cartilage

5. _____ is the term used to describe the accidental inhalation of liquids or solids into the lower airway. (C 2-1.7)

   a. regurgitation
   b. asphyxiation
   c. aspiration
   d. exsanguination

6. The bronchi divide into smaller airways until they communicate with the small air sacs with very thin walls that are surrounded by capillaries. These structures are called: (C 2-1.1)

   a. alveoli
   b. protein
   c. red blood cells
   d. tissues

7. Air in the pleural space is called a _____, and blood in this space is called a _____. (C 2-1.3)

   a. pericothorax, pneumothorax
   b. hemothorax, epithorax
   c. hemithorax, pneumothorax
   d. pneumothorax, hemothorax

8. Because of the smaller size of the chest wall, infants and children depend more heavily on the _____ for breathing. (C 2-1.2)

   a. accessory muscles
   b. diaphragm
   c. hypothalamus
   d. bronchiole

9. Nasal airways are less likely to stimulate the gag reflex than are oral airways. (C 2-1.17, 18)

   a. true
   b. false

10. The absence of breath sounds on one side of the chest in a patient who is acutely short of breath is a very serious sign. It can indicate: (C 2-1.3)

    a. impending respiratory failure
    b. transecting abdominal aneurysm
    c. impending congestive failure
    d. isolated head injury

11. The head-tilt–chin-lift maneuver is the easiest technique for opening an airway in patients without a suspected spinal injury. (C 2-1.4 and P 2-1.25)

    a. true
    b. false

12. When a cervical spine injury is suspected, the jaw thrust maneuver should be performed. The EMT kneels behind the supine patient with his or her hands stabilizing the patient's head and neck. While maintaining cervical immobilization, the EMT thrusts the jaw: (C 2-1.6 and P 2-1.26)

    a. forward
    b. downward
    c. backward
    d. sideways

13. A patient requires suctioning whenever: (C 2-1.8)

    a. other attempts to clear the airway fail
    b. a gurgling sound is heard during breathing
    c. fluid is seen in the airway of an unconscious patient
    d. all of the above

14. Suction is applied while withdrawing the catheter in a side-to-side motion for a maximum of __ seconds. (P 2-1.27)

   a. 20
   b. 15
   c. 10
   d. 25

15. The proper size oropharyngeal airway is selected by measuring from the: (C 2-1.17 and P 2-1.35)

   a. corner of the mouth to the angle of the jaw
   b. corner of the eye to the tip of the nose
   c. corner of the ear to the tip of the chin
   d. all of the above

16. The nasopharyngeal (nasal) airway is a semi-rigid device that can be inserted into the nose of patients who cannot tolerate an oropharyngeal airway. The proper size nasopharyngeal airway is selected by measuring from the: (C 2-1.18 and P 2-1.36)

   a. tip of the nose to the tip of the ear
   b. corner of the eye to the tip of the nose
   c. corner of the ear to the tip of the chin
   d. all of the above

17. Techniques used by EMTs for artificial ventilation include all of the following **except**: (C 2-1.9–15 and P 2-2.29)

   a. mouth-to-mask, two person BVM
   b. flow-restricted, oxygen-powered ventilator device
   c. one person BVM
   d. simple face mask, nonrebreather mask

18. Mouth-to-mask ventilation is the most effective method of artificial ventilation for a single rescuer. (C 2-1.9)

   a. true
   b. false

19. Increasing minute ventilation above normal is called: (C 2-1.10)

   a. hyperventilation
   b. hypoventilation
   c. hypooxygenation
   d. ventilation ratio

20. _____ is especially important in the management of patients with head injuries. (C 2-1.10)

   a. Hyperventilation
   b. Hypoventilation
   c. Hypooxygenation
   d. Ventilation ratio

21. The oxygen inlet and reservoir of the BVM allow for high concentrations of inspired oxygen at approximately: (P 2-1.31, 32)

   a. 40–90%
   b. 80–100%
   c. 45–70%
   d. 60–85%

22. The appropriate BVM for prehospital care use consists of all of the following **except**: (C 2-1.12 and P 2-1.30)

    a. face mask
    b. one-way valve
    c. self-inflating bag and oxygen reservoir
    d. pop-off valve

23. Because of the difficulty of maintaining an airtight seal while squeezing the bag, a single EMT should perform mouth-to-mask ventilation or use a flow-restricted oxygen-powered ventilator before using the BVM alone. (C 2-1.12)

    a. true
    b. false

24. When two EMTs are available, the BVM can be a very effective device. Both EMTs should: (C 2-1.12–14)

    a. kneel behind the patient's head and insert an oral or nasal airway
    b. watch for chest rise and listen for breath sounds to ensure adequate ventilation
    c. obtain an airtight mask seal with the same technique used for face mask application
    d. not concern themselves with air accumulating in the stomach

25. If a trauma patient requires artificial ventilation, a cervical spine injury is assumed until proven otherwise. (C 2-1.12)

    a. true
    b. false

26. Flow-restricted, oxygen-powered ventilators provide ____% oxygen at a maximum flow rate. (C 2-1.15)

    a. 40
    b. 60
    c. 80
    d. 100

27. Flow-restricted, oxygen-powered ventilators should only be used with: (P 2-1.33)

    a. adults
    b. adolescents
    c. neonates
    d. pediatrics

28. If no tracheostomy tube is present, the opening in the neck is referred to as a: (C 2-1.16 and P 2-1.34)

    a. gastrostomy
    b. stoma
    c. mouth
    d. barrier

29. When opening an infant's airway and administering oxygen, the neck should be kept in a _____ position. (P 2-1.40, 41)

    a. extended
    b. hyperextended
    c. neutral
    d. hyperflexed

30. Patients with a depressed level of consciousness and a respiratory rate of less than 12 or more than 24 breaths/min are likely to require assisted ventilations. (A 2-1.23, 24)

    (a) true
    b. false

31. Any cylinder that contains oxygen is _____ in color. (C 2-1.19)

    a. red
    (b) green
    c. brown
    d. black

32. Oxygen cylinders must be handled carefully since their contents are under very high pressure. The pressure of a full cylinder is approximately _____ psi (pounds per square inch). (C 2-1.19 and P 2-1.37)

    a. 1,000
    b. 5,000
    c. 3,000
    (d) 2,000

33. Nasal cannulas deliver a low concentration of oxygen. They should only be used in: (C 2-1.21 and P 2-1.39)

    a. unconscious patients who are in respiratory distress
    (b) stable patients who are not in acute respiratory distress
    c. stable patients who are in acute respiratory distress
    d. stable patients who present with chest pain

34. The maximum flow rate with the nasal cannula is: (C 2-1.22)

    (a) 5−6 L/min
    b. 8−10 L/min
    c. 2−4 L/min
    d. 10−12 L/min

35. Patients with acute respiratory distress should be given high concentrations of oxygen with a nonrebreather mask, even if they have a history of chronic obstructive pulmonary disease (COPD). (C 2-1.20 and P 2-1.38)

    (a) true
    b. false

36. The nonrebreather mask is the best method of providing high concentrations of supplemental oxygen to the spontaneously breathing prehospital patient. With high flow rates (15 L/min), the mask can deliver up to __% oxygen. (C 2-1.20)

    a. 20
    b. 40
    c. 60
    (d) 90

37. When administering CPR, a barrier device should be used: (P 2-1.28)

    (a) always
    b. never
    c. when dealing with nonemergent patients
    d. when dealing with a patient known to have tuberculosis

38. The symptom of shortness of breath is called: (C 2-1.3)

    a. eupnea
    b. orthopnea
    c. tachypnea
    d. dyspnea

Scenario

Read each scenario. Write the answers to the corresponding questions in the space provided.

SCENARIO #1:

Your EMT crew is called to the scene of a 60-year-old female patient who is found to be unresponsive. She is lying in bed. You note snoring and gurgling respirations. The patient's daughter informs you that her mother has a history of shortness of breath due to allergies. You notice that the patient is breathing through her mouth at a rate of 42 breaths/min and her respirations are shallow.

    As you are assessing the airway, your partner is checking the patient's blood pressure (B/P). As you complete your assessment of the airway your partner informs you that the B/P is within normal limits and the heart rate is 100 beats per minute (BPM).

1. What initial interventions will you perform?

    _____

    _____

    _____

    _____

2. How would you further manage this patient?

    _____

    _____

    _____

    _____

CHAPTER 11 ANSWERS TO REVIEW QUESTIONS

		8. b	**16.** d	**24.** a	**32.** d
		7. d	**15.** a	**23.** a	**31.** b
38. d	**6.** a	**14.** b	**22.** d	**30.** a
37. a	**5.** c	**13.** d	**21.** b	**29.** c
36. d	**4.** a	**12.** a	**20.** a	**28.** b
35. a	**3.** a	**11.** a	**19.** a	**27.** a
34. a	**2.** c	**10.** a	**18.** a	**26.** d
33. b	**1.** a	**9.** a	**17.** d	**25.** a

SCENARIO SOLUTIONS

Scenario #1:

1. This patient needs high concentration oxygen immediately. Upon arrival you should perform a head-tilt chin-lift, to open the airway and suction the patient, as needed.
2. Oxygen should be administered to this patient at 15 L/min. If the patient becomes unable to manage her respirations, you may assist respirations by giving artificial breaths with the patient's spontaneous breaths.

   An airway adjunct such as an oropharyngeal airway should be inserted if the patient has no gag reflex. Frequent vital sign checks should be made to make sure the patient does not require chest compressions.

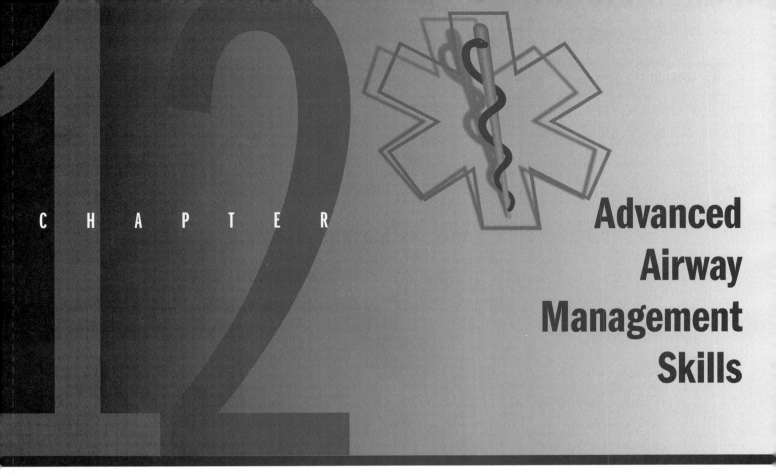

CHAPTER 12

Advanced Airway Management Skills

Reading Assignment: Chapter 12, pgs. 201–223

OBJECTIVES

1. Identify and describe the anatomical structures involved in performing endotracheal intubation in the adult, infant, and child.

2. Recognize and explain the pathophysiology of airway compromise, including the indications and rationale for advanced airway management by EMT-Bs.

3. Describe and demonstrate the techniques used for endotracheal intubation in the infant, child, and adult, which include choosing an appropriate size endotracheal tube, inserting a stylet, using both curved and straight blades for intubation, securing the endotracheal tube, and demonstrating endotracheal suctioning.

4. Describe and demonstrate the skill of confirming endotracheal tube placement, including the use of end-tidal carbon dioxide detection and/or other detection techniques.

5. Recognize the complications of advanced airway management, including the consequences of unrecognized esophageal intubation.

6. Recognize and respect the feelings of the patient and family regarding advanced directives as they apply to endotracheal intubation.

INTRODUCTION

Airway management is the first priority in both basic and advanced life support. The use of advanced airway management skills by the EMT-B is a new proposition aimed at improving patient outcomes. All EMTs who perform endotracheal intubation need thorough initial training, frequent practice, and close supervision in the classroom and in the field.

This chapter presents a review of anatomical structures, signs and symptoms of airway compromise and the indications for advanced airway management. In addition, this chapter describes endotracheal intubation skills for the infant, child, and adult.

This chapter is optional for EMT-B education. Although endotracheal intubation is the preferred airway for many critically ill or injured patients, ventilation takes priority over intubation.

REVIEW QUESTIONS

Please circle one correct answer for each question.

1. The mouth and nose are the beginning of the upper airway. The base of the tongue extends down to the: (C 8-1.1)

   a. epiglottis
   b. carina
   c. pharynx
   d. vallecula

2. The _____ is used as a landmark during endotracheal intubation. (C 8-1.1)

   a. turbinate
   b. carina
   c. pharynx
   d. vallecula

3. The _____ _____ protect the opening of the trachea from aspiration of liquids and foreign material. (C 8-1.1)

   a. front teeth
   b. vocal cords
   c. chordae tendineae
   d. nasal turbinates

4. The combination of a proportionally larger tongue and a smaller larynx makes the vocal cords appear more _____ in infants and children than in adults. (C 8-1.2)

   a. posterior
   b. anterior
   c. inferior
   d. superior

5. The EMT must be careful during intubation because the upper airway structures of infants and children are more rigid and less fragile than those of adults. (C 8-1.2)

   a. true
   b. false

6. The most common cause of an obstructed airway in an unconscious patient is the: (C 8-1.3)

   a. teeth
   b. mucus
   c. tongue
   d. epiglottis

7. Other causes of airway obstruction include: (C 8-1.3)

   a. respiratory secretions
   b. gastric contents and foreign bodies
   c. blood and teeth
   d. all of the above

8. The alveolar/capillary exchange cannot function properly when a patient has a(n): (C 8-1.3)

   a. obstructed airway
   b. endotracheal tube
   c. nasopharyngeal airway
   d. oropharyngeal airway

9. Prior to intubation, a patient should always be ventilated with BLS techniques. (C 8-1.4)

   a. true
   b. false

10. The immediate concern with a patient who has poor or absent respirations is: (C 8-1.3)

    a. hypoxia
    b. anemia
    c. tachypnea
    d. asphyxia

11. Endotracheal intubation is indicated when any of the following criteria exist **except**: (C 8-1.8)

    a. the patient is unresponsive to painful stimuli
    b. the patient has a gag reflex or is coughing
    c. the patient is unable to protect the airway
    d. the patient is in cardiac arrest

12. Body substance isolation techniques, including masks and protective eyewear, must be used whenever attempting endotracheal intubation. (C 8-1.9)

    a. true
    b. false

13. The _____ is the instrument used to visualize the vocal cords for endotracheal tube placement. (C 8-1.9)

    a. microscope
    b. laparoscope
    c. otoscope
    d. laryngoscope

14. Two primary blades are used for intubation: the curved blade and the straight blade. The curved blade is designed to be inserted into the: (C 8-1.10)

    a. vallecula
    b. epiglottis
    c. esophagus
    d. vocal cords

15. The straight blade is designed to lift the _____ directly during endotracheal intubation. (C 8-1.11)

    a. trachea
    b. carina
    c. epiglottis
    d. vocal cords

16. A stylet is used to: (C 8-1.12 and A 8-1.25)

    a. provide firmness to the endotracheal tube during insertion
    b. act as a guide for the laryngoscope blade
    c. insert nasopharyngeal airways
    d. target the carina

17. A stylet that protrudes from the end of the endotracheal tube can: (C 8-1.12)

    a. facilitate intubation attempts
    b. injure airway structures during insertion
    c. serve as a securing device for the endotracheal tube
    d. be used to eliminate the need for the oropharyngeal airway

18. When choosing the appropriate size endotracheal tube, the EMT should remember the emergency rule that states: (C 8-1.13)

    a. a 7.5-mm tube fits an adult
    b. a 4-mm tube fits an adult
    c. a 10-mm tube fits most males
    d. a 7-mm tube fits a small child

19. A curved blade is often preferred for intubating infants because of better tongue displacement and vocal cord visualization. (P 8-1.31)

    a. true
    b. false

20. A formula that is useful for selecting endotracheal tube size in children is to add 16 plus the age in years and divide by: (C 8-1.14)

    a. 6
    b. 4
    c. 2
    d. 3

21. Another method for estimating endotracheal tube size is to use the size of: (C 8-1.16)

    a. the infant's little finger
    b. your little finger
    c. the infant's thumb
    d. the infant's index finger

22. In children less than _ years old, an uncuffed endotracheal tube is used. (C 8-1.9)

   a. 9
   b. 12
   c. 16
   d. 8

23. Endotracheal intubation allows complete control of the airway and is the definitive airway management technique. The most critical and potentially fatal complication of this procedure is: (C 8-1.15, 20 and A 8-1.23, 27)

   a. trauma to the pharynx
   b. esophageal intubation
   c. trauma to the lips and teeth
   d. hyperventilation

24. A second life-threatening complication of endotracheal intubation is that prolonged unsuccessful attempts lead to inadequate oxygenation. To avoid this complication, the EMT should limit any single attempt to: (C 8-1.17 and 18)

   a. 30 seconds
   b. 60 seconds
   c. 45 seconds
   d. 15 seconds

25. A single EMT should not attempt to intubate a patient more than twice. Before each attempt the patient must be hyperventilated with ___ oxygen to provide adequate preoxygenation. (C 8-1.5 and P 8-1.30)

   a. 80%
   b. 90%
   c. 100%
   d. 125%

26. It must be emphasized that the priority for an apneic patient is ventilation, not intubation. (C 8-1.17, 18)

   a. true
   b. false

27. It is important to monitor vital signs before and after the endotracheal intubation procedure because: (C 8-1.15)

   a. endotracheal intubation can change the heart rate
   b. during intubation the heart rate remains constant
   c. the patient may become hypothermic during the procedure
   d. the patient may vomit during the procedure

28. Once the tube is properly positioned, it must be appropriately secured in place to avoid accidental: (C 8-1.21, A 8-1.28, P 8-1.34, 35)

   a. extubation
   b. hyperperfusion
   c. hyperventilation
   d. hypotension

29. The only true way of confirming that the endotracheal tube enters the trachea is by: (C 8-1.19)

    a. visualizing the tube as it passes through the pharynx
    b. listening to lung sound on the right
    c. visualizing the tube as it passes between the vocal cords
    d. auscultate over the epicardium

30. A nasogastric tube (NG tube) is used for: (C 8-1.6)

    a. stomach decompression
    b. medication administration
    c. nutrition and/or gastric lavage
    d. all of the above

31. An absolute contraindication for NG tube placement is: (C 8-1.6)

    a. the presence of major facial trauma
    b. the possibility of a gastric ulcer
    c. the presence of major abdominal injury
    d. an open pneumothorax

32. To insert an NG tube, the patient is placed in a _____ position with the head turned to the ____ side. (C 8-1.6)

    a. prone, right
    b. supine, left
    c. prone, left
    d. supine, right

33. The Sellick maneuver can be used to help prevent passive regurgitation and aspiration during endotracheal intubation. This maneuver involves applying pressure to the: (C 8-1.7 and P 8-1.29)

    a. cricoid cartilage
    b. hyoid cartilage
    c. pleural cartilage
    d. vocal cords

34. Many patients have living wills that specify the interventions they wish to receive in the event of an emergency such as cardiac arrest. If there is **ANY** question about what the patient's wishes are, the EMT should: (A 8-1.22)

    a. attempt to perform all the interventions that are indicated for proper patient care
    b. not ask to see the actual document that outlines what the patient wants
    c. respect the patient's wishes and leave the scene immediately
    d. perform the interventions after consulting with the family clergy

35. Methods frequently used to check ET tube placement include all of the following **except**: (P 8-1.32 and 33)

    a. carbon dioxide detectors
    b. observing chest rise and fall
    c. listen to right and left apex
    d. auscultate over the epicardium

Scenarios

Read each scenario. Write the answers to the corresponding questions in the space provided.

SCENARIO #1:

Your first week at the new county ambulance service is about to come to an end. Thus far, the week has been rather uneventful. When you lie down for the night, you are making plans for the upcoming fourth of July weekend. The next thing you know the tone goes off and you and your crew are en route to the scene of an MVA involving an 18-year-old male. He is the only patient injured in the accident.

When you gain access to the patient, you note that the patient is not breathing and has a bluish tint to his lips and nailbeds. The patient is assessed as a "U" on the AVPU scale. Your partner informs you that the patient's pulse is 124, rapid and thready.

1. What immediate basic life support skills are required to manage this patient's airway?

_____

_____

_____

_____

2. What are the indications for advanced airway management?

_____

_____

_____

_____

3. Are there any contraindications to endotracheal intubation in this patient?

_____

_____

_____

_____

continued

SCENARIO # 2:
You and your EMT partner are providing EMS coverage at a local music park when you are called to the scene of a 6-year-old female patient who has fallen off the back of a pickup truck. When you arrive, the patient has been moved by bystanders to the side of the road. The patient is responsive only to painful stimuli. You note that the patient's respirations are 6 per minute and shallow. En route to the hospital, the patient ceases to breathe.

1. What are your initial actions at the scene?

_____

_____

_____

_____

2. How would you manage the patient when she becomes apneic?

_____

_____

_____

_____

CHAPTER 12 ANSWERS TO REVIEW QUESTIONS

1. a	**8.** a	**15.** c	**22.** d	**29.** c
2. d	**9.** a	**16.** a	**23.** b	**30.** d
3. b	**10.** a	**17.** b	**24.** a	**31.** a
4. b	**11.** b	**18.** a	**25.** c	**32.** b
5. b	**12.** a	**19.** b	**26.** a	**33.** a
6. c	**13.** d	**20.** b	**27.** a	**34.** a
7. d	**14.** a	**21.** a	**28.** a	**35.** d

SCENARIOS SOLUTIONS

Scenario #1:

1. Immediate BLS interventions should include:
   a. C-spine stabilization
   b. clearing the airway
   c. inserting an oropharyngeal airway
   d. the patient requires artificial ventilation with 100% oxygen using a technique such as BVM ventilation
2. The indications for advanced airway management in this patient include apnea, unresponsiveness, and the mechanism of injury (i.e., MVA with trauma). This patient clearly cannot control his own airway. The definitive airway in this patient is an endotracheal tube.
3. The contraindications for endotracheal intubation are negligible in this patient. If the patient becomes responsive (i.e., develops a gag reflex), endotracheal intubation by the EMT-B would not be indicated.

1. Immediate interventions should include:
   a. C-spine stabilization
   b. clearing the airway
   c. inserting an oropharyngeal airway
   d. the patient requires artificial ventilation with 100% oxygen using a technique such as BVM ventilation
2. Management of this patient's apnea includes:
   a. vigorous hyperventilation with 100% oxygen
   b. endotracheal intubation, with proper tube and blade sizes being carefully considered

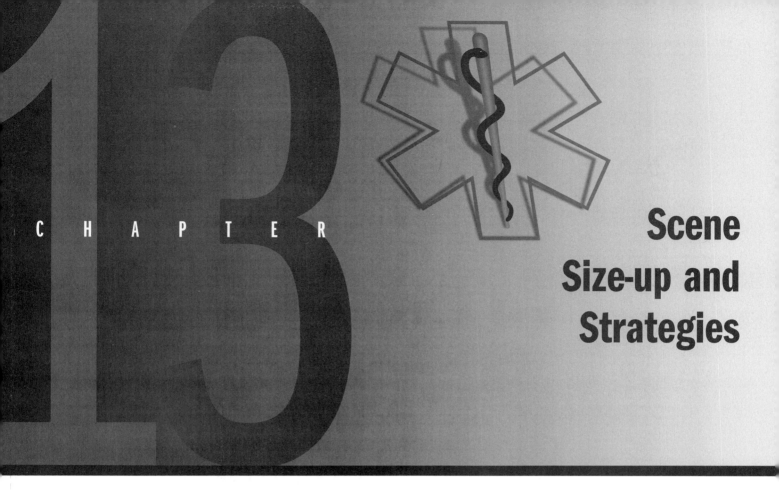

Scene Size-up and Strategies

CHAPTER 13

Reading Assignment: Chapter 13, pgs. 224–235

OBJECTIVES

1. Describe the importance of scene evaluation, both while en route to and on arrival at the scene, and the impact on the outcome of the patient.

2. Describe emergency medical dispatch and its role in helping the EMT develop strategies for delivery of the best possible patient care.

3. Describe the key elements of the scene survey, gained from both the dispatcher and the survey of the scene on arrival, that can impact the outcome of patient care.

4. Describe the potential threat hazardous materials present to both the EMT and the patient at the scene of a medical emergency.

5. Describe the necessary safety measures to be taken for protection of both the patient and EMTs at a scene.

6. Describe the importance of personal protective equipment to the EMT's safety and reduction of contamination by blood-borne pathogens or other potentially infectious materials in caring for a patient.

7. Describe how bio-ethical considerations affect the resuscitation of patients in the prehospital setting.

8. Rapidly assess the appropriateness of a DNR order and describe how it is used to implement or withhold resuscitation.

9. Rapidly assess the appropriateness of a living will and describe how it is used to implement or withhold resuscitation.

10. Rapidly assess the appropriateness of an advance directive and describe how it is used to implement or withhold resuscitation.

11. Rapidly assess the appropriateness of a durable power of attorney and describe how it is used to implement or withhold resuscitation.

INTRODUCTION

The development of and improvements in emergency medical dispatch have improved EMS response. This chapter discusses the design of dispatch, which ensures that the EMS unit receives pertinent information to initiate scene management upon arrival.

The EMT must be knowledgeable of concepts that may affect the management of a scene as well as the delivery of patient care. The scene must be assessed rapidly for risks that may be present. The EMTs must then quickly ensure their own safety and determine appropriate actions to ensure that neither the patient nor rescuers become exposed unnecessarily to increased risk.

Evaluation of the scene is a critical component of patient care. Emergency medical technicians should not enter unsafe scenes, and should be aware of community resources that can provide assistance.

REVIEW QUESTIONS

Please circle one correct answer for each question.

1. Which of the following elements are part of the scene survey? (C 3-1.5)

   a. number of patients
   b. hazards or potential hazards that exist
   c. need for additional resources
   d. need to cancel additional resources that have been dispatched and are not needed

   1. 1, 3
   2. 2, 3
   3. 1, 2, 3, 4
   4. 3, 4

2. Different hazards can be present that pose a threat to the safety of the EMT. Upon arriving at a scene, which type of call can present the greatest number of risks to the EMT? (C 3-1.1)

   a. medical
   b. trauma
   c. obstetric
   d. nontrauma

3. Evaluation of the mechanism of injury can assist with: (C 3-1.4)

   a. determining the number of patients that are involved
   b. evaluating the patient(s) for possible injuries
   c. determining the need for initiating resuscitation
   d. all of the above

4. It is important for EMTs to review the dispatch information while en route to a call because it will help to ensure that the most appropriate care can be given in the shortest time frame. Another reason is: (C 3-1.7)

   a. to cancel any unneeded resources that were dispatched
   b. to assure their own safety
   c. to provide a complete and comprehensive radio report
   d. to identify reasons not to transport the patient(s)

5. Scene hazards may include: (C 3-1.2)

   a. downed power lines
   b. broken gas transmission lines
   c. toxic substances that have been spilled
   d. all of the above

6. Depending upon the completeness of the caller's description, dispatch information enables the EMT to determine whether the call: (C 3-1.6)

   a. is a trauma or medical call
   b. includes any life-threatening conditions
   c. involves fire, building or other hazards
   d. all of the above

7. Scene size-up is: (C 3-1.3)

   a. the best way to reduce exposure to communicable diseases
   b. a rapid assessment of the scene and scene surroundings
   c. a decision regarding priority of patient care
   d. triage

8. When you arrive at a scene involving hazardous materials, your highest priority is: (C 3-1.1)

   a. personal safety
   b. patient safety
   c. public safety
   d. triage

9. Upon arrival at a scene involving multiple vehicles, the EMT must consider: (C 3-1.5)

   a. that more medical personnel may be needed on the scene
   b. whether helicopter evacuation is a possibility
   c. whether the scene requires special equipment
   d. all of the above

10. If the weather is very hot or very cold, the medical condition of the patient may be aggravated and treatment plans altered to avoid unnecessary exposure to the elements. (P 3-1.9)

    a. true
    b. false

11. Emergency medical technicians should never enter a scene involving reported violence until he or she confirms that the scene is secure. (C 3-1.3)

    a. true
    b. false

12. Hazardous materials are transported on commercial carriers and are a regular part of EMS scene response and management. All hazardous materials should be considered a threat to the EMT until proven otherwise. (C 3-1.1)

    a. true
    b. false

13. When approaching the scene, a critical clue for determining the possible injuries that a patient may have sustained at a trauma call is/are the: (C 3-1.4)

    a. patient's symptoms
    b. bystanders' reactions
    c. time of the call
    d. mechanism of injury

14. The EMT must quickly evaluate the total scene at a trauma call to help determine the probable mechanism of injury. At the scene of a motor vehicle collision this evaluation involves: (C 3-1.4)

    a. determining how the vehicle(s) collided
    b. approximating the speed involved at the time of impact
    c. whether safety belts were used to restrain the victims
    d. all of the above

15. At an industrial accident, evaluation might include: (C 3-1.4)

    a. the height that the victim fell
    b. the amount of debris that fell on the victim
    c. the type of machinery involved in the accident
    d. all of the above

16. When considering safety concerns the EMT should remember that any scene that involves the threat of violence should be controlled by the: (C 3-1.7)

    a. human resources department
    b. police department
    c. fire department
    d. EMS department

17. The presence of a physician on the scene dictates that: (A 3-1.8)

    a. the call will always be a frustrating situation
    b. the situation will require tact on the part of the EMT
    c. the physician identify his or her presence and show identification
    d. both b and c

18. The physician should be informed that the scene is under the control of the medical control physician. The EMT should then: (A 3-1.8)

   a. establish interface between medical control and the physician at the scene
   b. assure that all care is being directed by the on-scene physician
   c. disregard protocols that have been approved by the authority in the community
   d. allow the on-scene physician to provide the medical care of the patient

19. Compassion for the patient and his or her family is demonstrated by: (A 3-1.8)

   a. actions
   b. words
   c. mannerisms
   d. a, b, and c

20. Personal Protective Equipment (PPE) is designed to protect emergency personnel from the risk of contamination by: (C 3-1.2)

   a. blood
   b. airborne contaminants
   c. other potentially infectious materials
   d. all of the above

21. Personal Protective Equipment includes full face protection and gloves when dealing with any situation where you could be at risk from blood or other potentially infectious materials. (C 3-1.2)

   a. true
   b. false

22. One definition of a multiple casualty incident is "any scene that involves": (C 3-1.5)

   a. one or more victims
   b. a pediatric patient
   c. conditions that the responding unit cannot handle
   d. multiple patients who do not present with obvious injuries

23. Triage is: (C 3-1.5)

   a. the sorting and allocation of treatment to patients to maximize the number of survivors
   b. accomplished by stopping at the first patient and beginning treatment
   c. preventing the involvement of bystander assistance
   d. the performance of life-saving interventions

24. Do Not Resuscitate legislation is designed to give patients the opportunity to express their wishes in writing concerning resuscitation efforts and to give prehospital care providers the legal parameters to follow these resuscitation decisions. (A 3-1.8)

   a. true
   b. false

25. Initial scene evaluation is necessary to determine the need for additional resources and/or the presence of a hazardous material. (C 3-1.3)

a. true
b. false

Scenario

Read each scenario. Write the answers to the corresponding questions in the space provided.

SCENARIO #1:

You are the lead EMT on the EMS unit today and thus far it has been an uneventful day. It is 10:00 AM on a Monday morning. You and your partner are dispatched to an automobile accident with injuries. A van has careened off the road into a ditch. En route to the scene the dispatcher advises you that one vehicle is involved, with unknown numbers of patients and injuries.

Upon arrival at the scene you notice smoke coming from the back of the van. The brush adjacent to the van is on fire. The accident occurred in sight of the local fire department and they are in the process of extinguishing the fire. You observe an adult female patient climbing from a vehicle and you hear the driver crying out that he cannot move his legs.

1. What steps would you take while traveling to the scene?

_____

_____

_____

_____

2. Upon arrival, what will be your initial priorities and steps of management?

_____

_____

_____

_____

3. How many victims were involved in this accident?

_____

_____

_____

_____

CHAPTER 13 ANSWERS TO REVIEW QUESTIONS

1. c	**6.** d	**11.** a	**16.** b	**21.** a
2. b	**7.** b	**12.** a	**17.** d	**22.** c
3. d	**8.** a	**13.** d	**18.** a	**23.** a
4. b	**9.** d	**14.** d	**19.** d	**24.** a
5. d	**10.** a	**15.** d	**20.** d	**25.** a

7. The initial access and ongoing communications that occur between the EMT in the field and the physician at the hospital are the keys to minimizing transport delay. (A 3-7.10)

   a. true
   b. false

8. Which of the following areas allow for the most rapid EMS response times? (Chp. #14, Obj. #1)

   a. urban
   b. sparsely populated
   c. wilderness
   d. rural

9. In areas where dispatchers are trained specifically to give prearrival instructions, one of the key decisions confronting the dispatchers is the: (C 3-7.8)

   a. patient's age
   b. receiving hospital
   c. logistics
   d. level of care required

10. After receiving the dispatch order from the EMD, the EMT should obtain as much information as possible to help prepare for the scene. Examples of the types of information that may be helpful include: (C 3-7.1)

    a. type of call
    b. age and sex of the patient
    c. location of the incident
    d. all of the above

11. All of the following are priorities of scene management **except**: (C 3-1.5)

    a. equipment most likely needed
    b. type insurance the patient maintains
    c. the roles of each member of the team
    d. treatment procedures that will be required

12. As the ambulance pulls up to the scene, the first consideration is the: (C 3-1.3)

    a. personal safety of the crew
    b. patient locality
    c. bystander security
    d. extrication procedures

13. Scene control may be the responsibility of: (C 3-1.3)

    a. police
    b. fire personnel
    c. EMS personnel
    d. all of the above

14. The original dispatch information should: (C 3-7.9)

    a. bias your conclusions
    b. create tunnel vision
    c. complement the findings presented
    d. determine patient care priorities

15. If the scene situation and the patient's condition permit, the EMT should first: (C 3-7.7)

    a. communicate directly with the patient
    b. talk with first responders
    c. talk with friends and coworkers
    d. speak with relatives who are present on the scene

16. Upon entering the scene, an EMT must take notice of the surroundings and the factors that will positively or negatively impact the ability to work effectively. (C 3-3.1)

    a. true
    b. false

17. A critical component of being an EMT and responding to an EMS call involves the ability to take command of the situation. _____ is the ability to influence others to carry out assigned tasks and to perform as required according to those assignments. (Chp. # 14, Obj. #7)

    a. Dictatorship
    b. Leadership
    c. Control
    d. Monopoly

18. In an emergency situation, the need to delegate authority is critical for all of the following to occur, **except:** (Chp. # 14, Obj. #7)

    a. directives to be carried out
    b. each member of the team to understand his or her assignment
    c. medical control interaction
    d. patient care delivery

19. The purpose of effective communication is: (C 3-7.3)

    a. to transmit information
    b. to avoid communication with the family and bystanders
    c. to avoid written reports
    d. to negate the need for additional directives

20. All pertinent information (data) gathered by the EMT during the various phases of assessment must be documented and communicated to the: (P 3-7.12)

    a. county health department
    b. human resources division
    c. emergency department staff
    d. law enforcement agency

21. The method of transportation should be considered as soon as: (C 3-2.1)

    a. enough information is gathered
    b. the crew arrives at the scene
    c. life-threatening conditions are managed
    d. a and c

22. Choosing one hospital over another depends primarily upon: (C 3-2.19)

    a. patient request
    b. proximity and specialized care availability
    c. emergency department patient diversion status
    d. local protocols

23. To ensure continuity of care, it is important that the EMT remain with the patient throughout the transfer process in the emergency department. (C 3-7.1)

    a. true
    b. false

24. It is imperative that all findings be documented on the prehospital care report (PCR). In the medical profession, it is generally accepted that "what has not been documented on the PCR is assumed not to have been done." (C 3-7.6)

    a. true
    b. false

25. A total EMS system includes: C 1-1.1)

    a. first responders
    b. BLS units
    c. advanced life support units
    d. all of the above

Scenarios

Read each scenario. Write the answers to the corresponding questions in the space provided.

SCENARIO #1:

Your crew is dispatched to a stabbing at a local pool hall. Dispatch informs you that there are two victims involved in the dispute.

1. List at least five questions you should consider.

_____

_____

_____

_____

_____

SCENARIO #2:

A wakeup call at 2:00 AM dispatches you and your EMT crew to the scene of a motor vehicle crash involving three vehicles. Several questions should go through your mind while en route to the scene.

1. List at least ten questions that you and your crew should consider.

_____

_____

_____

_____

CHAPTER 14 ANSWERS TO REVIEW QUESTIONS

1.	a	**6.**	a	**11.**	b	**16.**	a	**21.**	d
2.	b	**7.**	a	**12.**	a	**17.**	b	**22.**	d
3.	b	**8.**	a	**13.**	d	**18.**	d	**23.**	a
4.	c	**9.**	d	**14.**	c	**19.**	a	**24.**	a
5.	d	**10.**	d	**15.**	a	**20.**	c	**25.**	d

SCENARIOS SOLUTIONS

Scenario #1:

1. Questions to consider would include:
   - Has the area been secured by law enforcement?
   - Do the patients have a single or multiple wound(s)?
   - Is more than one patient present?
   - Who are the good guys and the bad guys?
   - Where are the weapons?
   - What BSI precautions should be undertaken?

Scenario #2:

1. Questions to consider would include:
   - What problems may be encountered?
   - Will there be any hazards to me or my partner?
   - Who has been identified as the team leader for this call?
   - What will need to be done first?
   - On surveying the situation what is noticed?
   - What are the priorities when beginning to treat the patients?
   - Can the situation be handled with the available resources?
   - Which ED should be the destination hospital?
   - Has the area been appropriately marked with safety lights/flares?
   - Are flammable liquids present?
   - Does this incident involve hazardous materials?
   - Is law enforcement on the scene?
   - Is the fire department on the scene?

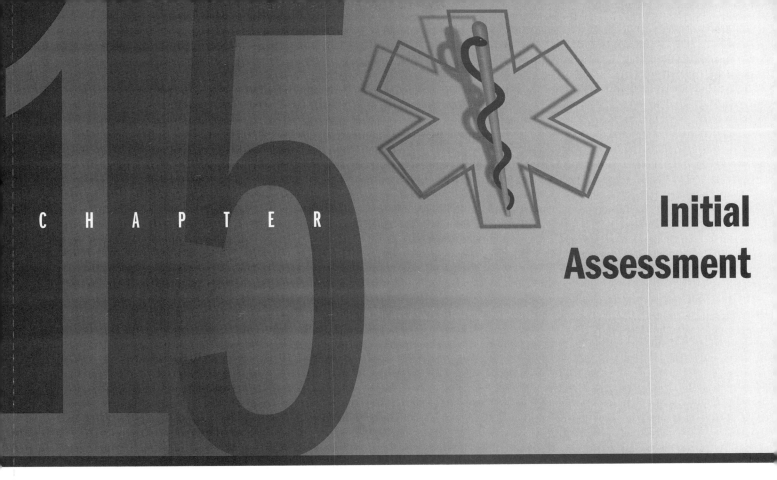

C H A P T E R

Initial
Assessment

Reading Assignment: Chapter 15, pgs. 250−282

OBJECTIVES

1. Differentiate between safe and unsafe scenes.

2. Demonstrate the ability to handle the situation appropriately.

3. Understand the concept of an assessment-based approach to patient care.

4. Understand the reason for and the timing of interventions.

5. Understand that interventions may include specific patient care, transportation, or further assessment.

6. Describe and demonstrate the various parts of a complete assessment including scene size-up, initial assessment, rapid, focused history and physical exam, detailed physical exam, and ongoing assessment.

7. Perform an appropriate, real time, patient assessment and identify the need for appropriate interventions, in real time as well as in simulated situations.

8. Demonstrate the completion of the patient assessment, as appropriate, during transportation.

INTRODUCTION

Assessment is a critical component of EMT skills that must be mastered through practice, experience, and ongoing evaluation. Assessment and interventions must be tailored to the individual patient and circumstances. The actions of the EMT must be dictated by the condition of the patient.

The EMT must continually assess the patient and provide necessary interventions based upon the initial assessment findings. These interventions must be consistent with the knowledge and skill level of the healthcare provider at the scene.

This chapter provides information about the various stages of assessment, including: scene size-up; initial assessment; rapid, trauma- or medical-focused history and physical examination (medical and trauma); detailed physical examination; and ongoing assessment.

REVIEW QUESTIONS

Please circle one correct answer for each question.

1. The objective of the rapid, focused history and physical exam is to discover any potential life-threatening condition. (C 3-2.1)
   a. true
   b. false

2. The correct order for performing the first three steps of initial patient assessment is: (C 3-2.19)
   a. initial assessment, scene size-up, ongoing assessment
   b. scene size-up, initial assessment, detailed physical examination
   c. scene size-up, initial assessment, rapid, focused history and physical examination
   d. initial assessment, rapid, focused history and physical examination, scene size-up

3. Triage is: (C 3-2.20)
   a. a thorough inventory of the available equipment on the unit
   b. the process of sorting patients to determine which ones require immediate treatment and transport
   c. a French word meaning "to sort"
   d. b and c

4. Once the general impression is formed, it never changes throughout the survey. (3-2.1)
   a. true
   b. false

5. Upon entering a scene and finding a patient who is sitting forward in a chair, pale, sweating, and struggling to breathe, the EMT forms an initial impression of an individual with breathing difficulty and begins to formulate a plan of action. The 'plan of action' might include: (3-2.1)
   a. the need for administration of oxygen
   b. transporting the patient in a sitting position
   c. preparing for possible complications such as airway problems
   d. all of the above

6. To quickly determine the patient's level of consciousness or responsiveness, the EMT should use the: (C 3-2.2)

    a. APGAR system
    b. SAMPLE history
    c. AVPU system
    d. PRQST system

7. When assessing the mental status of an adult patient, you note that the patient does not respond until you apply a painful stimulus. This patient's level of consciousness is best indicated by the letter: (C 3-2.3)

    a. A - alert
    b. V - responds to verbal stimuli
    c. P - responds to painful stimuli
    d. U - unresponsive

8. When dealing with trauma patients with an altered level of consciousness or mechanism of injury indication, a high level of suspicion of cervical spinal injury should be maintained. (C 3-2.5)

    a. true
    b. false

9. To check the level of consciousness in a 6-month-old infant who appears drowsy, the EMT should: (C 3-2.3)

    a. shake the infant by his arms
    b. perform a sternal rub
    c. gently pat the baby on his head
    d. tap the bottom of the feet

10. If at any point during the assessment, the EMT determines that the patient is a priority or that attempted life-saving interventions are not working, transportation and ALS activation should be initiated immediately while assessments and interventions are continued en route. (C 3-2.19)

    a. true
    b. false

11. The adequacy of the patient's breathing may be assessed rapidly by: (C 3-2.4)

    a. listening to the chest
    b. looking at the chest
    c. feeling the chest
    d. all of the above

12. Airway problems require immediate interventions. If an intervention does not work: (C 3-2.8)

    a. the general impression should be reevaluated
    b. prompt transportation must be considered
    c. triage should be employed
    d. the medical control physician should be called to the scene

13. When evaluating an unconscious patient, one reliable way to assess breathing is to: (C 3-2.6)

    a. check the pulse
    b. check for capillary refill
    c. check for chest rise and fall
    d. assess the blood pressure

14. Initial assessment of a 16-year-old diabetic patient reveals adequate breathing. Based on this finding, the EMT should: (C 3-2.7)

   a. immediately transport the patient
   b. observe the patient while continuing the initial assessment
   c. assist respiration with a BVM
   d. ventilate the patient without supplemental oxygen

15. In an unresponsive patient or a patient with a decreased level of consciousness who is breathing, but not adequately, the EMT must also assist the patient's respirations. Assisted ventilations can be accomplished by: (C 3-2.11)

   a. mouth-to-mask
   b. BVM
   c. flow-restricted, oxygen-powered ventilation device
   d. all of the above

16. When distinguishing between methods of assessing breathing in the adult, child and infant one thing to remember is: (C 3-2.10)

   a. the respiratory rates will be within the same ranges
   b. the child patient normally breathes faster than the infant
   c. the infant breathes faster than the adult patient
   d. the range for the adult patient is 24–30 breaths/min

17. The airway of the adult nontrauma patient should be opened by the rescuer's placing one hand on the forehead and the other hand: (C 3-2.11)

   a. on the larynx
   b. under the chin
   c. above the neck
   d. under the neck

18. The presence or absence of a pulse is determined by feeling for a radial pulse at either wrist. If a pulse cannot be felt, the _____ artery in the ____ should be checked. (C 3-2.12)

   a. carotid, neck
   b. brachial, arm
   c. femoral, leg
   d. radial, neck

19. If a patient is one year old or less, feel for the _____ pulse in the ____. (C 3-2.13)

   a. carotid, neck
   b. brachial, arm
   c. femoral, leg
   d. radial, neck

20. The absence of a pulse without other signs of death is a clue to: (C 3-2.13)

   a. check the pulse in another location
   b. contact the coroner
   c. have a family member check it
   d. notify the nearby ALS units

21. If major external bleeding is evident, the EMT should initially control the bleeding with: (C 3-2.14)

   a. direct pressure
   b. pressure point
   c. pressure dressing
   d. tourniquet

22. In reference to Question #21, if bleeding cannot be controlled with this intervention: (C 3-2.14)

   a. immediate transportation should be initiated
   b. immediate endotracheal intubation should be initiated
   c. ALS should be called, if available
   d. pressure dressing should be employed

23. Adequate _____ means that oxygenated blood is getting to all of the tissues and organs of the body. (A 3-2.21)

   a. perfusion
   b. bleeding
   c. pulse
   d. temperature

24. Internal bleeding and poor perfusion are suspected based on: (C 3-2.15)

   a. the mechanism of injury
   b. nature of illness
   c. assessment findings such as pale skin color
   d. all of the above

25. Capillary refilling may be less useful in adults than for infants and children. (C 3-2.18)

   a. true
   b. false

26. If a patient is exhibiting no signs of shock, the EMT would expect the skin condition to reveal: (C 3-2.17)

   a. contusion and ecchymosis
   b. warmth and dryness to touch, pink color
   c. coolness to touch
   d. dryness and coolness to touch

27. Cool, clammy extremities may indicate: (C 3-2.16)

   a. poor perfusion
   b. hypothermia
   c. hyperthermia
   d. hypertension

28. The purpose of the ongoing assessment is to: (C 3-2.19)

   a. reassess the patient for changes that may require new interventions
   b. look for omissions, and evaluate the effectiveness of earlier interventions
   c. reassess earlier significant findings
   d. all of the above

29. Critical patients should be reassessed: (C 3-2.21)

   a. every 4 minutes
   b. frequently
   c. only at the scene
   d. once, during transport

30. The ongoing assessment is continued until the patient is: (C 3-2.21)

   a. transferred to the ALS unit
   b. transferred to a higher level of care
   c. discharged from the definitive care facility
   d. showing signs of improvement

Scenarios

Read each scenario. Write the answers to the corresponding questions in the space provided.

SCENARIO #1:

It's been a busy Friday night thus far, and it's only 10:00 PM when the emergency phone line rings. The dispatcher supplies you with the following information:

Respond to 124 Mill Street to assist a 65-year-old female who awoke suddenly complaining of difficulty breathing. You and your partner are immediately en route to the scene, when additional information is provided by the dispatcher: the patient's neighbor reports that the patient awoke about 10 minutes ago and called her for help. She is sitting in her bedroom and is having trouble breathing. She has no history of this type illness.

1. Why should you form a general impression?

_____

_____

_____

_____

2. When should you and your partner begin putting a plan of action together?

_____

_____

_____

_____

3. What would be your plan of action?

_____

_____

_____

_____

continued

SCENARIO #2:

Your BLS ambulance is dispatched to a motor vehicle crash involving eight victims. While en route, the EMTs learn that two vehicles are involved and some of the victims may be trapped.

1. With this information, what should the EMT's plan of action regarding backup include?

_____

_____

_____

_____

On arrival at the scene, it is noted that the scene is secure. One patient is trapped in the vehicle and is in serious condition. The other seven patients have visible injuries.

2. What is the proper term for the process by which identification of the most serious patients is performed?

_____

_____

_____

_____

CHAPTER 15 ANSWERS TO REVIEW QUESTIONS

1. a	7. c	13. c	19. b	25. a
2. c	8. a	14. b	20. a	26. b
3. d	9. d	15. d	21. a	27. a
4. b	10. a	16. c	22. d	28. d
5. d	11. d	17. b	23. a	29. b
6. c	12. b	18. a	24. d	30. b

SCENARIOS SOLUTIONS

Scenario #1

1. The general impression is formed to determine priority of care and is based on the EMT's immediate assessment of the environment and the patient's chief complaint. Without going through the process of forming a general impression and developing a plan of action, onscene time may be prolonged. Time is lost and the patient could also be lost while deciding what actions to take. Remember, both the general impression and plan of action are, and should be, adjusted as more information becomes available.

2. Your initial plan of action should be constructed around the dispatch information while en route to the scene. It should be adjusted as more information becomes available.

3. The dispatch information is valuable and informative enough to assist you in beginning to formulate your plan of action. Generally scenes such as this are safe. Your plan of action should include:

   a. Assuring scene safety and personal safety.

b. Entering the house with oxygen, stretcher, and basic jump kit containing a blood pressure cuff, airways, and appropriate airway equipment.

c. Perform an initial assessment to determine onset of symptoms and adequacy of breathing, circulation, or both.

d. Initiate supplemental oxygen administration, assess baseline vital signs (pulse, B/P).

e. Transport the patient to a definitive care facility, remembering to contact an ALS unit if available.

Scenario #2

1. The EMT should request assistance from additional ambulance units, the fire and police departments, and an ALS helicopter unit, if available. Extrication personnel should be mobilized.

2. Triage.

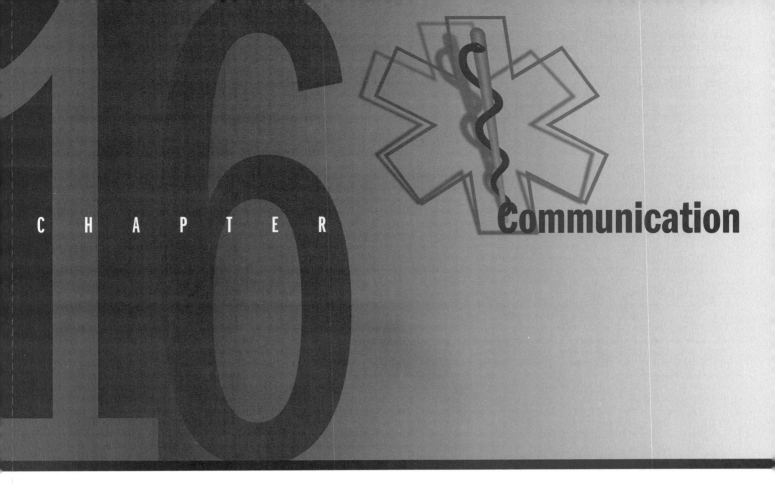

CHAPTER 16

Communication

Reading Assignment: Chapter 16, pgs. 283–298

OBJECTIVES

1. Describe the importance of communication in an EMS system.

2. Identify the components of an EMS communication system.

3. Describe the various methods available to the public to access the EMS system.

4. Explain the principles of emergency medical dispatch.

5. Describe the process for dispatching EMS agencies, including the use of computer-aided dispatch.

6. Demonstrate appropriate use of radio communication with the dispatch center in various phases of an ambulance call.

7. Describe the role of radio communication between the EMT and medical direction.

8. Identify the essential components and proper sequence of delivery of an oral patient report.

INTRODUCTION

This chapter describes the basic components of an EMS communication system. It includes the characterization of each system component and describes important principles of use. Effective communication skills are essential in the medical profession. The ability to communicate clearly and efficiently is necessary in every component of the EMS system.

Essential components of EMS communications include access to the system, methods of dispatching, communication with medical control and EMT/patient communications. The EMT must also be able to communicate with patient's families.

Effective communication skills are some of the most important that an EMT must learn. This chapter provides the basic information necessary to successfully master this topic.

REVIEW QUESTIONS

Please circle one correct answer for each question.

1. The type of radio installed in the ambulance is called a: (C 3-7.1)
    a. base station
    b. mobile unit
    c. portable unit
    d. manual unit

2. A device that receives a low-power transmission and retransmits the signal at higher power is called a: (C 3-7.1)
    a. remote station
    b. base station
    c. repeater
    d. beeper

3. A radio that is located at a stationary site such as a hospital, mountain top, or public safety agency is called a: (C 3-7.1)
    a. repeater
    b. base station
    c. mobile radio
    d. portable radio

4. Emergency Medical Services systems are moving away from the use of codes because of the possibility of miscommunication. The simplest way to make sure that everyone understands what is being said is to: (C 3-7.3)
    a. communicate in plain English
    b. utilize only written communications
    c. speak softly into the microphone
    d. speak rapidly in a soft tone

5. All of the following are reasons that prehospital personnel need to communicate with the hospital **except**: (C 3-7.3)

 a. to communicate with a physician
 b. to receive medical direction
 c. to provide the emergency department with notice of the patient's arrival so that initial preparations can begin
 d. to explain your diagnosis of the patient's condition

6. When considering the proper sequence for delivery of patient information, which items that follow should be stated first when calling the hospital? (C 3-7.2)

 a. B/P = 140/100
 b. patient is allergic to penicillin
 c. 65-year-old male
 d. history of asthma

7. Mobile radios are radios that are mounted in vehicles such as ambulances or fire engines. Mobile radios are much less powerful than portable radios. (A 3-7.10)

 a. true
 b. false

8. The center of the communication system is called the _____ _____, and employs a special group of people called dispatchers to receive calls for assistance and dispatch emergency personnel and vehicles. (C 3-7.5)

 a. dispatch facility
 b. incident command
 c. command center
 d. mobile transmitter

9. Public access to an EMS system is influenced by a number of factors, including: (C 3-7.8)

 a. capability of local telephone company equipment
 b. public service budgets of local and regional governments
 c. competition within single political jurisdictions over control of public access
 d. all of the above

10. The most common method for accessing the EMS system is the: (C 3-7.8)

 a. telephone
 b. roadside call boxes
 c. E 911 system
 d. repeater

11. General principles of radio use include all of the following **except**: (C 3-7.1)

 a. make sure that the radio is turned on and properly adjusted
 b. listen to the frequency to make sure that there is no other traffic before transmitting
 c. speak clearly and distinctly
 d. press the talk switch on the microphone and wait 10 seconds

12. Prenotification of the patient's arrival to the receiving hospital can dramatically reduce the time interval between arrival at the emergency department and initiation of definitive treatment. (A 3-7.10)

    a. true
    b. false

13. The essential elements of a radio report to the receiving facility include: (C 3-7.4)

    a. identify unit and level of provider
    b. estimated time of arrival (ETA)
    c. age and sex of the patient
    d. all of the above

14. A brief description of the symptoms of which the patient is complaining is called the: (C 3-7.4)

    a. chief symptom
    b. primary complaint
    c. chief complaint
    d. diagnosis

15. Emergency Medical Services personnel should notify the dispatcher as soon as the unit leaves the scene with the patient. This notification informs the dispatcher that: (C 3-7.9)

    a. the unit is back in service and ready for another call
    b. work on the scene is concluded and transport has begun
    c. the patient's condition has improved
    d. all of the above

16. While en route, the EMT continues to assess and provide care for the patient. Any significant change in patient condition or response to treatment should be reported to the receiving facility. (C 3-7.9)

    a. true
    b. false

17. As the patient is delivered to the receiving hospital, the EMT must report verbally to hospital personnel. It is appropriate for the EMT to turn responsibility for a patient over to any of the following individuals **except**: (C 3-7.9)

    a. physician
    b. registered nurse
    c. licensed practical nurse
    d. admissions clerk

18. General principles of interpersonal communication include all of the following **except**: (C 3-7.7)

    a. act and speak in a calm and confident manner
    b. do not maintain eye contact with the patient
    c. speak clearly, slowly, and distinctly
    d. treat the patient with respect

19. When dealing with hearing-impaired patients, the EMT should: (C 3-7.7)

   a. always speak clearly with lips clearly visible to the patient
   b. learn basic sign language to help him or her communicate
   c. exchange written notes with the patient
   d. all of the above

20. All of the following are responsibilities of the Federal Communication Commission (FCC) **except**: (C 3-7.6)

   a. approval of radio frequencies
   b. monitoring radio frequencies
   c. licensing and allocation of radio frequencies
   d. allocating funds for the purchase of radios

Scenarios

Read each scenario. Write the answers to the corresponding questions in the space provided.

SCENARIO #1:

It is a busy night at the local base hospital emergency room (ER). You and your partner arrive with your patient who responds only to verbal stimuli. Your partner is assisting the patient's ventilations with a BVM. Every member of the hospital ER staff is busy with other emergent patients and no one can stop to take your report at the present time.

1. What should you and your crew do in this situation?

_____

_____

_____

_____

SCENARIO #2:

You and your crew are called to the residence of an elderly couple at approximately midnight. The wife meets you at the door, appearing very flustered. She is weeping and tells you that her husband, who is 76 years of age, has undergone two bypass surgeries in the past 2 years and that he just awoke from sleep complaining of severe chest pain.

   Upon entering the bedroom, you find an elderly gentleman sitting up in the bed, clutching his nightshirt. He is perspiring profusely and you note that his skin is ashen. He denies shortness of breath. Initial assessment demonstrates that the patient's B/P is 180/96, pulse is 66 and regular, and respirations are 24 and somewhat labored. You note no jugular vein distention and his breath sounds are clear bilaterally. You elect to administer oxygen via nonrebreather mask at a rate of 15 L/min.

1. List the proper sequence for delivery of patient information when calling the hospital in reference to this patient.

_____

_____

_____

_____

CHAPTER 16 ANSWERS TO REVIEW QUESTIONS

1.	b	**5.**	d	**9.**	d	**13.**	d	**17.**	d
2.	c	**6.**	c	**10.**	a	**14.**	c	**18.**	b
3.	b	**7.**	b	**11.**	d	**15.**	b	**19.**	d
4.	a	**8.**	a	**12.**	a	**16.**	a	**20.**	d

SCENARIOS SOLUTIONS

Scenario #1:

1. You must stay with your patient until the time that there can be an orderly transfer of responsibility to qualified emergency department medical personnel. Your patient clearly has a need for continuing care and remains your responsibility until such time that a qualified ER staff member can receive your verbal and written report and assume responsibility for the patient.

Scenario #2:

1. The patient is a 76-year-old male who called for an ambulance because of severe chest pain. The pain woke him from sleep a few minutes prior to the call for help. He denies shortness of breath. The patient has a history of recent cardiovascular surgery. Patient has no history of allergies.

   On physical examination, he is found to be perspiring profusely, and his skin is ashen in color.

   His vital signs are as follows: B/P is 180/96, pulse is 66 and regular, and respirations are 24 and somewhat labored. There is no jugular venous distention and lung sounds are clear bilaterally.

   Oxygen is being administered at 15 L/min via nonrebreather mask.

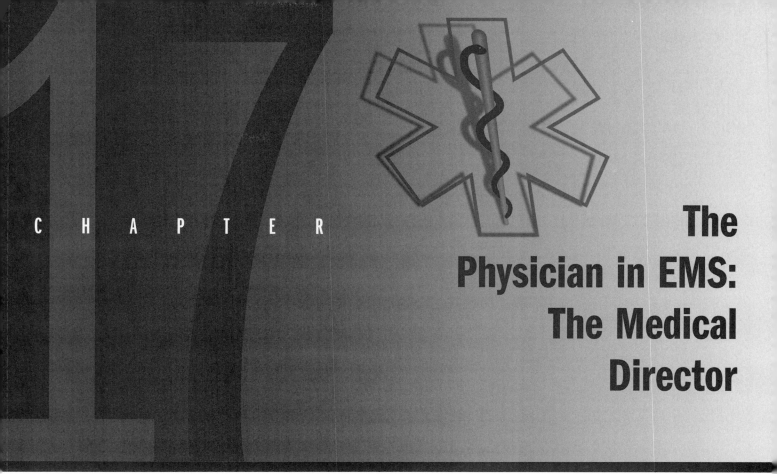

The Physician in EMS: The Medical Director

Reading Assignment: Chapter 17, pgs. 299–310

OBJECTIVES

1. Describe the roles and responsibilities of the EMS medical director.

2. Identify three approaches to EMS medical direction.

3. List the components of prospective medical direction.

4. Identify the components of immediate medical direction.

5. List the components of retrospective medical direction.

6. Explain the importance of the relationship between the EMT and the medical director.

INTRODUCTION

The relationship between the physician and the prehospital provider has its foundation in history, theory, and law. An accepted healthcare delivery principle is that quality patient care results from the cooperative efforts of many different providers.

The modern EMS model is designed to take emergency medical care out of the hospital and to the patient, and thereby reduce the amount of time between onset of the illness, injury, or both and the initiation of emergency care. Emergency medical services were implemented through the use of physician extenders who were specially trained individuals prepared to act as the physician's eyes, ears, and hands in the prehospital evaluation and management of the emergency patient. These physician extenders became known as EMTs.

To implement the physician extender concept, prehospital emergency care providers were given authority to deliver healthcare through appropriate state laws or regulations. Through medical practice laws, the responsibility for EMT practice was placed on the physician who agreed to supervise the prehospital providers. In this chapter, EMS medical direction, roles and responsibilities of the physician in the EMS system, and the relationship between the medical director and the EMT are addressed.

REVIEW QUESTIONS

Please circle one correct answer for each question.

1. The three approaches to medical direction discussed in this chapter include all of the following **except**: (C 1-1.6)

   a. prospective medical direction
   b. immediate medical direction
   c. retrospective medical direction
   d. proactive medical direction

2. The EMT-B curriculum strongly recommends that even the most basic EMS service have a medical director. (C 1-1.6)

   a. true
   b. false

3. _____ describe the entire evaluation and treatment process for a particular presenting symptom or chief complaint. (C 1-1.6)

   a. Standing orders
   b. Protocols
   c. Guidelines
   d. Recommendations

4. Medical direction of EMS systems is standardized in all states. (C 1-1.6)

   a. true
   b. false

5. Medical direction at its most basic level means that paramedics determine what emergency medical care is provided in an EMS system and spell out exactly how the care will be provided. (C 1-1.6)

   a. true
   b. false

6. Prospective medical direction includes the range of activities that a medical director may be involved with that occur _____ the time that the emergency occurs. (C 1-1.6)

   a. before
   b. after
   c. during
   d. near

7. The medical director can have a major impact on the care provided in a system by being actively involved in all of the following activities **except**: (C 1-1.6)

    a. training the providers in the system
    b. identifying the equipment that will be used to treat patients
    c. being responsible for daily maintenance of the vehicles
    d. assisting with selection of personnel

8. Immediate medical direction includes the range of activities that a medical director provides: (C 1-1.6)

    a. while the emergency is actually taking place
    b. before the emergency actually takes place
    c. after the emergency takes place
    d. during the 6-month period before the unit is licensed

9. _____ describes the activities conducted by the physician after the call is complete. (C 1-1.6)

    a. Prospective medical direction
    b. Immediate medical direction
    c. Retrospective medical direction
    d. Proactive medical direction

10. The EMS medical director must be involved in two different types of activities to accomplish the three approaches to medical direction. The first type of activities are administrative in nature and are known as: (C 1-1.6)

    a. offline medical direction
    b. indirect medical direction
    c. direct medical direction
    d. a and b

11. Offline medical direction includes activities such as: (C 1-1.6)

    a. writing protocols
    b. reviewing EMT performance
    c. other administrative duties
    d. all of the above

12. The second type of activities for the EMS medical director are clinical in nature. This clinical type of medical direction is also known as: (C 1-1.6)

    a. online medical direction
    b. indirect medical direction
    c. offline medical direction
    d. executive medical direction

13. Online medical direction activities may include: (C 1-1.6)

    a. providing radio or telephone instructions to prehospital providers
    b. direct observation of system and individual performance
    c. in some systems, responding to the scene and providing prehospital patient care
    d. all of the above

14. The _____ is the responsible authority for healthcare delivery, including prehospital patient care. (C 1-1.6)

    a. governor
    b. paramedic
    c. physician
    d. hospital administrator

15. Emergency Medical Services medical direction is recognized as a specialized set of knowledge and skills. (C 1-1.6)

    a. true
    b. false

16. The physician who provides medical direction for an EMS system should possess all of the following characteristics **except**: (C 1-1.6)

    a. familiarity with the design and operation of prehospital EMS systems
    b. a state license as an EMT-Paramedic that certifies that the physician has completed an advanced level EMS course
    c. experience in prehospital emergency care of the acutely ill or injured patient
    d. knowledge of base-station radio control of prehospital emergency units

17. It is a desirable aspect of prehospital care that the EMS medical director should maintain active involvement in the training of basic and advanced life support prehospital personnel. (C 1-1.6)

    a. true
    b. false

18. The prospective phase of EMS medical direction begins when: (C 1-1.6)

    a. a community first makes the decision to provide EMS service
    b. a community identifies the type of EMS vehicles that they want to purchase
    c. a community spells out the resources and limitations on system design
    d. a and c

19. While the administrative entities that provide the financial support for EMS services have concerns and responsibilities, the factors that impact the quality of medical care must ultimately be the responsibility of the _____. (C 1-1.6)

    a. governor
    b. paramedic
    c. physician
    d. hospital administrator

20. Protocol approval may come from a: (C 1-1.6)

    a. state government agency
    b. local government agency
    c. state medical organization
    d. all of the above

21. The goal of the protocol approval process is to assure that: (C 1-1.6)

  a. the medical community agrees with the proposed level of prehospital care
  b. the proposed level of care and protocols accurately reflect the standard of care in the community
  c. communitywide medical personnel supports the prehospital system
  d. all of the above

22. With information now available about the effectiveness of standing orders, many EMS systems are shifting away from requirements for direct, online medical direction and, instead, focusing more on the use of standing orders. (C 1-1.6)

  a. true
  b. false

23. As experience continues to build, it is becoming clear that the key to the success of a standing orders-based system is the presence of an effective: (C 1-1.6)

  a. indirect medical direction process
  b. clinical medical direction process
  c. direct medical direction process
  d. online medical direction process

24. Protocols developed by the medical director will influence training in the system. (C 1-1.6)

  a. true
  b. false

25. Physicians can be an excellent resource for some aspects of the EMT training program. These aspects include: (C 1-1.6)

  a. classroom participation that provides an opportunity for EMTs to get to know the medical director
  b. physician involvement in the actual presentation of training
  c. the medical director's contributions to the continuing education program for the EMS system
  d. all of the above

26. A list of basic equipment and supplies for an ambulance that identifies standard equipment necessary to provide adequate patient care at the basic, intermediate, and advanced levels has been identified by the: (C 1-1.6)

  a. American Academy of Pediatric Surgeons
  b. American College of Family Practitioners
  c. American College of Surgeons/Committee on Trauma
  d. American College of Orthopedic Physicians

27. The key to ambulance placement, dispatch, hospital communication, and immediate review of the current status of the EMS system is the: (C 1-1.6)

  a. communication component
  b. run review component
  c. prospective component
  d. transportation component

28. The physician who provides direct (online) medical direction may or may not be the same physician who has responsibility for the administrative, prospective, or retrospective aspects of an EMS system's medical control. (C 1-1.6)

    a. true
    b. false

29. Retrospective medical direction is also known as: (C 1-1.6)

    a. quality assurance
    b. prospective analysis
    c. respective direction
    d. retrospective critique

30. The EMS medical director should be involved in the routine review of the emergency medical calls handled by the EMS system. The purpose of this review is: (C 1-1.6)

    a. to identify systemwide issues such as response time or skill problems that affect everyone
    b. to identify individual providers who may have specific educational needs
    c. to involve the physician looking at the patient care report that was prepared by the EMTs, as well as the hospital records for the patient if they are available
    d. all of the above

Scenario

Read each scenario. Write the answers to the corresponding questions in the space provided.

SCENARIO #1:

You and your EMT crew are enjoying your 24-hour shift more than usual at your ambulance company. Today, one of the ER physicians who provides medical direction for your ambulance service is riding on the ambulance with you for 8 hours. It has been a slow day thus far, with only two routine transfers to be handled during the shift.

Your crew and the physician have spent the morning reviewing patient care reports. At 12 noon, the dispatcher sends you and your EMS personnel to the scene of a motor vehicle accident. The dispatcher also sends rescue and fire crews. Upon arrival at the scene, you notice that one car is involved in the MVA with two victims visible at the scene size-up. The patients are rapidly evaluated, treated, and transported to the local receiving hospital.

At the hospital, the online medical director, the physician who is riding with you, and you and your crew review the events leading up to delivery of the patient to the hospital. After you have completed the patient care report, you again discuss the care that the patient received.

It is now 2 PM and you and your crew return to the station, leaving your special guest at the hospital since his shift with you has ended and his shift at the ER begins at 3 PM.

1. Which of the approaches to medical direction were used in this scenario?

    _____

    _____

    _____

    _____

continued

2. List at least four advantages that the EMT crew realized by having the physician ride with them during this shift.

    _____

    _____

    _____

    _____

3. Which types of medical direction were used in this scenario?

    _____

    _____

    _____

    _____

CHAPTER 17 ANSWERS TO REVIEW QUESTIONS

30. d	24. a	18. d	12. a	6. a
29. a	23. a	17. a	11. d	5. b
28. a	22. a	16. b	10. d	4. b
27. a	21. d	15. d	9. c	3. b
26. c	20. d	14. c	8. a	2. a
25. d	19. c	13. d	7. c	1. d

SCENARIO SOLUTIONS

Scenario #1

1. The prospective medical, immediate, and retrospective medical direction approaches were used.

2. The advantages are as follows:
    - a physician was onscene to provide medical care
    - a physician provided both direct and indirect medical direction for the EMS service
    - the ER physician had the opportunity to work with the EMTs to assure that the system was medically and administratively sound
    - the EMTs' training and skill levels could be evaluated at an actual scene
    - the end result is that patients received high quality patient care with direct physician involvement

3. The types of medical direction were online (direct) and offline (indirect).

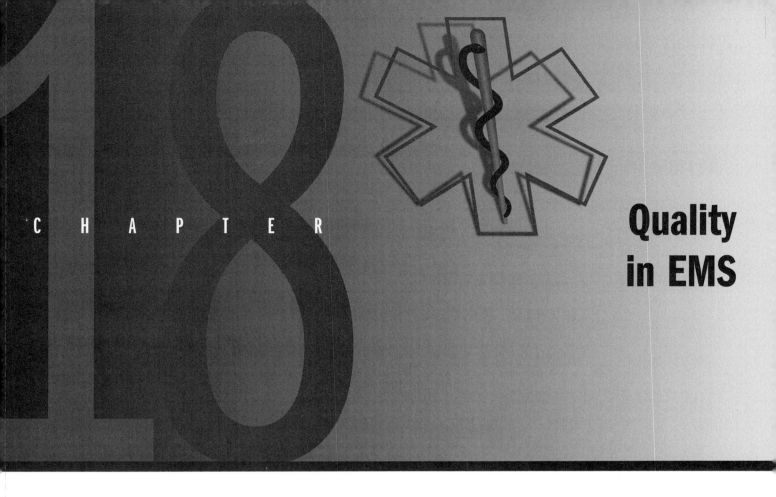

Quality in EMS

Reading Assignment: Chapter 18, pgs. 311–319

OBJECTIVES

1. Define quality assurance (QA) and continuous quality improvement (CQI).

2. Define the following terms as they apply to QA:
   - Prospective evaluation
   - Concurrent evaluation
   - Retrospective evaluation

3. Describe four methods used in a continuous quality improvement program in which an EMT is likely to become involved.

INTRODUCTION

Quality is a vital issue in the healthcare system. Synonymous with quality is the word excellence. It is the EMT's responsibility to understand and apply the principles of quality emergency medical care. Improvement in patient care is the ultimate goal for the QA program.

These principles begin with the care provided to the sick or injured and include collecting data, evaluation of the care provided (both from the perspective of process and outcome), and utilization of the knowledge concepts learned through study and experience. This chapter introduces the basic concepts of quality measurement and evaluation and reviews the basic components of a QA program.

REVIEW QUESTIONS

Please circle one correct answer for each question.

1. An example of a prospective form of quality evaluation would be: (C 1-1.5)

   a. patient care report (PCR)
   b. physician riding with the ambulance crew
   c. skills check off
   d. online medical direction

2. An example of a retrospective form of quality evaluation would be: (C 1-1.5)

   a. PCR review
   b. physician riding with the ambulance crew
   c. skills check off
   d. online medical direction

3. Types of evaluation used to measure quality include all of the following **except**: (C 1-1.5)

   a. retrospective
   b. PCR review
   c. complaint investigation
   d. recurrent

4. Methods of CQI with which the EMT may become involved include: (C 1-1.5)

   a. data collection
   b. case reviews
   c. continuing education
   d. all of the above

5. Quality assurance is defined as a mix of activities designed to evaluate how well the EMS system and EMTs take care of patients. (C 1-1.5)

   a. true
   b. false

6. System performance is measured in a variety of ways to determine if care is delivered in a timely, efficient and medically sensible manner. The methods of measurement include evaluation of all of the following **except**: (C 1-1.5)

   a. response times
   b. patient survival
   c. skills proficiency
   d. salaries and benefits

7. Important aspects of QA include evaluating all of the following **except**: (C 1-1.5)

   a. training
   b. performance
   c. patient care
   d. cross training

8. Continuous quality improvement differs from QA in that it strives to continuously improve how the system takes care of patients. (C 1-1.5)

   a. true
   b. false

9. Examples of CQI include: (C 1-1.5)

   a. improving the quality of continuing education
   b. updating treatment protocols
   c. skills evaluation and remediation
   d. all of the above

10. Quality assurance measures system or individual performance against a certain standard, whereas CQI uses evaluation to continuously improve the EMS system. (C 1-1.5)

    a. true
    b. false

11. The individuals involved in both QA and CQI are important to an effective EMS system and the development of good patient care skills by the EMT. These individuals include the: (C 1-1.5)

    a. medical director
    b. EMTs
    c. ER staff
    d. all of the above

12. The basic methods available to medical directors to evaluate quality of EMT performance include all of the following **except**: (C 1-1.5)

    a. prospective
    b. concurrent
    c. retrospective
    d. preactive

13. Prospective evaluation tools are designed to improve the care delivered by the EMS system: (C 1-1.5)

    a. prior to responding to a call
    b. while responding to a call
    c. after responding to a call
    d. while delivering patient care

14. The prospective type of evaluation is generally thought to be the most valuable because it allows care to be improved before the emergency call takes place. (C 1-1.5)

    a. true
    b. false

15. Medical directors should have input into decisions concerning continuing education topics, equipment that should be carried, and hiring of personnel, as these issues can affect the quality of care. (C 1-1.5)

    a. true
    b. false

16. Concurrent evaluation in CQI programs includes: (C 1-1.5)

    a. the direct observation of care delivered by the EMT
    b. a physician providing online medical control
    c. medical director "ride alongs" with the EMT to observe patient care delivered in the field
    d. all of the above

17. Concurrent evaluation is the most useful kind of evaluation to the: (C 1-1.5)

    a. medical director
    b. dispatcher
    c. hospital administrator
    d. ER staff

18. Retrospective evaluation includes methods that are applied: (C 1-1.5)

    a. after an EMT has completed a call
    b. while the EMT is receiving the call
    c. before the EMT completes the call
    d. while the EMT is delivering patient care

19. Retrospective methods of evaluation are the most commonly used because of: (C 1-1.5)

    a. ease
    b. cost
    c. convenience
    d. all of the above

20. Which of the following methods may medical directors use to review what happened after an EMS call? (C 1-1.5)

    a. chart audits
    b. case reviews
    c. debriefings
    d. all of the above

21. Quality improvement loops are used to assure that quality is: (C 1-1.5)

    a. not measured
    b. marginally improved
    c. measured and improved
    d. measured annually

22. EMTs become involved in the quality improvement loop as: (C 1-1.5)

    a. data collectors
    b. valuable participants in the analysis phase
    c. the subjects of change (either in training or individual performance)
    d. all of the above

23. A good CQI program can assist the EMT in providing excellent patient care. (C 1-1.5)

a. true
b. false

24. The most important tools in data collection are the: (C 1-1.5)

a. medical directors
b. EMTs
c. patients
d. ER nurses

25. A method that helps the EMT identify the aspects of patient care that are important to the medical director is the: (C 1-1.5)

a. peer review
b. continuing education
c. case review
d. trends review

Scenario

Read each scenario. Write the answers to the corresponding questions in the space provided.

SCENARIO #1:

You are the EMT in charge of the shift today. John, one of your new EMTs, has reported to you that he is experiencing unusual difficulty with a specific skill: blood pressure measurement. As luck would have it, you have scheduled your monthly continuing education program this month to focus on vital sign assessment. Your medical director, Dr. Beard, is expected to arrive at the station within the next 30 minutes.

Just as the program begins, you and your crew receive a call to a residence. The chief complaint is reported as "dizziness." Dr. Beard elects to ride along with you on this call. You have briefed the doctor about your new crew member's problem with blood pressure readings.

Upon arrival at the scene, you find that the patient is alert and oriented and is in no distress. You and Dr. Beard elect to observe the new EMT while he gathers the vital sign data. After he has attempted to take the patient's blood pressure, you check after him and note that the blood pressure reading that you obtain differs significantly from the reading that your new crew member had noted.

At this time, you complete the patient assessment and transport the patient to the hospital. Upon arrival back at the station, Dr. Beard announces that he is very pleased with the quality of care that your crew has delivered to the patient. He then continues the session by reviewing the call that your crew just completed.

The followup review to this case reveals that the new EMT was overlooking the importance of correct stethoscope placement during the vital sign assessment. Dr. Beard elects to review the proper procedure for blood pressure assessment and begins the second part of the session by pairing the EMTs to go through vital sign skill sessions. Dr. Beard oversees the stations and works directly with your new EMT. He enjoys teaching and working with all the EMTs at the service.

At the end of the review session, Dr. Beard is pleased with your new partner's performance and you feel that this has been an excellent learning experience for all your crew members.

continued

1. What type of quality evaluation methods are being used in this scenario?

   _____

   _____

   _____

   _____

2. What benefits do you, your crew and your medical director receive from this type of activity?

   _____

   _____

   _____

   _____

3. How is patient care improved by this type of activity?

   _____

   _____

   _____

   _____

CHAPTER 18 ANSWERS TO REVIEW QUESTIONS

1. c	**6.** d	**11.** d	**16.** d	**21.** c
2. a	**7.** d	**12.** d	**17.** a	**22.** d
3. d	**8.** a	**13.** a	**18.** a	**23.** a
4. d	**9.** d	**14.** a	**19.** d	**24.** b
5. a	**10.** a	**15.** a	**20.** d	**25.** c

SCENARIO SOLUTIONS

Scenario #1:

1. In the scenario, the types of quality evaluation that are used include prospective, concurrent, and retrospective. Identifying and addressing a weakness in an EMT's skills before an EMS call is considered a prospective quality evaluation method. This method is very valuable when the medical director participates because the EMT learns first hand what the physician expects when it comes to patient care. Evaluating the EMT skills during patient care is considered a concurrent evaluation method, and reviewing the call is considered a retrospective quality evaluation method.

2. Both the medical director, you, and your crew benefit a great deal from this prospective evaluation. The medical director has the opportunity to observe first hand what type of care you and your crew are likely to deliver as well as to evaluate identified weaknesses.

3. Patient care is improved through the application of the prospective, concurrent and retrospective evaluation methods. Emergency medical technician skills are evaluated and improved. The physician demonstrates how the EMTs can improve their care based on evaluation of their skills, and this process establishes a quality improvement loop.

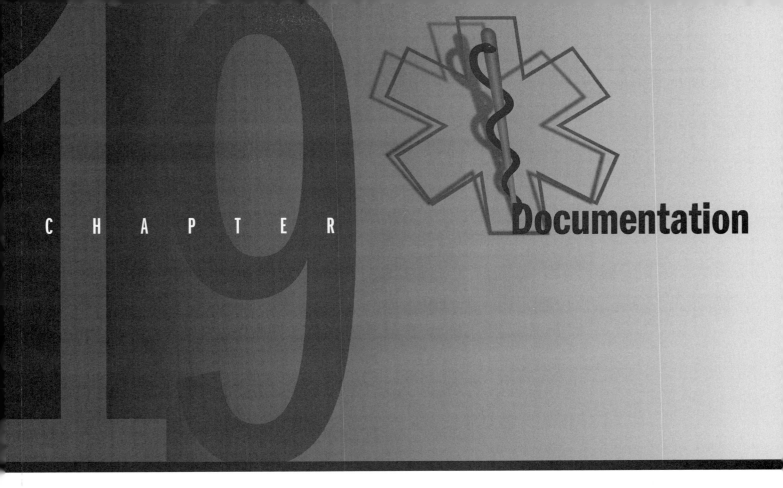

CHAPTER 19

Documentation

Reading Assignment: Chapter 19, pgs. 320–333

OBJECTIVES

1. Explain the importance of accurate documentation and report of patient care information.

2. List, explain, and apply the components of essential patient information in a written report.

3. Identify the various divisions of the written report.

4. Describe the information required in each section of the patient care report and how it should be entered.

5. Describe the legal implications associated with the written report.

6. State the proper sequence of delivery of patient information.

7. Define the special considerations concerning patient refusal.

8. Discuss all state and/or local record and reporting requirements.

9. Explain the purpose of gathering and reporting information.

INTRODUCTION

The patient care report documents the patient care delivered by the EMS crew in the prehospital setting. It is a confidential, legal document and may become a part of the patient's hospital record. An accurate and complete prehospital care report is important.

Should the care of the patient ever be called into question, the prehospital care record will be the EMT's first line of defense. Prehospital care reports are also used in quality improvement review, reimbursement, and for statistical review. This chapter will present several documentation guidelines as well as the division and sequence of the prehospital care report.

REVIEW QUESTIONS

Please circle one correct answer for each question.

1. A patient care report includes: (C 3-8.2)

   a. response data
   b. patient data
   c. narrative
   d. all of the above

2. The PCR is the official documentation of the physical assessment and treatment of a particular patient. (C 3-8.5)

   a. true
   b. false

3. The response data used for statistical analysis typically consist of all the following **except**: (C 3-8.3)

   a. patient name and date of birth
   b. service name and crew names
   c. unit number and mileage
   d. location of the call and crew license numbers

4. The patient data include which of the following? (C 3-8.3)

   a. the patient's name and home address
   b. date of birth and sex
   c. age and nature of call
   d. all of the above

5. The narrative section is provided for the EMT to document observations at the scene, assessment findings, and care and treatment delivered by the EMS crew. (C 3-8.1)

   a. true
   b. false

6. If a space on the PCR does not apply to the patient, you should: (3-8.3)

   a. mark it N/A
   b. leave it blank
   c. print your initials in it
   d. put a question mark in it

7. The patient care report should document the care delivered to the patient: (C 3-8.3)

    a. at the scene
    b. en route to the hospital
    c. medical care prior to the arrival of the EMS
    d. all of the above

8. The prehospital care report includes: (C 3-8.3)

    a. the patient's name, address, age, and sex
    b. the location of the emergency scene
    c. the findings of the assessment
    d. all of the above

9. Blank spaces in a prehospital care report lead the reader to believe that the report is not thorough or complete because information seems to be missing. (A 3-8.7)

    a. true
    b. false

10. In a patient complaining of abdominal pain, finding that the abdomen is soft and nontender to palpation is a: (C 3-8.3)

    a. pertinent negative
    b. pertinent positive
    c. insignificant finding
    d. false finding

11. When writing the narrative, the EMT should: (A 3-8.9)

    a. use slang terms and abbreviations
    b. approximate spelling when possible
    c. use plain language and correct spellings
    d. use "10 codes" only in the narrative

12. The initials SOAP mean: (C 3-8.2)

    a. subjective, objective, assessment, plan
    b. sensitive, objective, assessment, plan
    c. subjective, objective, assessment, patient
    d. subjective, offensive, assessment, patient

13. The head-to-toe method of documentation includes all of the following **except**: (C 3-8.2)

    a. the patient's age, sex, LOC, and initial presentation
    b. the results of your initial and focused assessments
    c. the treatment and care delivered
    d. the name of the family physician

14. Documentation based on the chronological progress of the call usually begins with the time of arrival on the scene. (C 3-8.2)

    a. true
    b. false

15. If a mistake is made while writing the narrative or on any part of the PCR, you should: (C 3-8.6)

    a. erase the mistake and continue the report
    b. mark out the mistake and continue the report
    c. draw a single line through the error and then place your initials beside the line and continue the report
    d. use correction fluid to cover the mistake and continue the report

16. When a mistake is discovered following the completion and/or submission of the report, the EMT should: (C 3-8.6)

    a. draw a single line through the error
    b. draw a double line through the error
    c. add a note with the correct information
    d. ask your partner to initial your error

17. In the event that information was omitted from a prehospital care report, the EMT should: (C 3-8.6)

    a. add a note with the information, the current date, and the EMT's initials
    b. should not be concerned about the omission
    c. make the correction to the report
    d. make a mental note if the report may be used later

18. When an error in patient treatment occurs, the EMT should: (C 3-8.6)

    a. try to cover up the mistake and not worry
    b. document what did or did not happen and the corrective action taken
    c. falsify the patient care report
    d. all of the above

19. Laws regarding confidentiality vary from state to state, so it is important for the EMT to familiarize himself or herself with the laws in his or her respective state. (C 3-8.6)

    a. true
    b. false

20. The EMT must ensure that the patient refusing care is: (C 3-8.4)

    a. able to make a rational, informed decision
    b. not under the influence of drugs or alcohol
    c. not under the effects of an illness or injury
    d. all of the above

21. If a patient refuses care, the patient should be: (C 3-8.4)

    a. encouraged to accept care
    b. informed why he or she needs to go to the hospital
    c. informed of what may happen if he or she does not accept care
    d. all of the above

22. When documenting the refusal situation, the EMT should include in the narrative: (C 3-8.4)

    a. complete patient assessment including vital signs
    b. the care that the EMS crew offered to provide
    c. that the patient was advised of possible consequences of refusing care and alternative care options
    d. all of the above

23. The narrative of a prehospital care report can be written using all of the following **except**: (C 3-8.2)

    a. using the SOAP method
    b. using head-to-toe method
    c. chronological order
    d. using the AVPU method

24. The initial S in SOAP refers to: (C 3-8.2)

    a. the treatment delivered by the EMT
    b. what the patient tells the EMT about his or her condition
    c. what the EMT observes about the patient
    d. the patient's overall condition

25. If the patient continues to refuse care, the EMT should do all of the following **except**: (C 3-8.4)

    a. have the patient sign a refusal form
    b. have the form signed by a witness
    c. contact medical control, if required by local policy
    d. leave the scene without the refusal form being signed

Scenario

Read each scenario. Write the answers to the corresponding questions in the space provided.

SCENARIO #1:
You and your partner arrive on the scene of a possible murder. The police have secured the scene. You approach the patient. The patient has a gunshot wound in the upper right back. The patient is breathing and has a pulse. You decide the patient is critical and call for immediate transport.

1. List at least six items that should be documented in the prehospital care report:

   _____

   _____

   _____

   _____

   _____

   _____

CHAPTER 19 ANSWERS TO REVIEW QUESTIONS

25. d	20. d	15. c	10. a	5. a
24. b	19. a	14. a	9. a	4. d
23. d	18. b	13. d	8. d	3. a
22. d	17. a	12. a	7. d	2. a
21. d	16. c	11. c	6. a	1. d

SCENARIO SOLUTIONS

Scenario #1:

1. The prehospital report should consist of the following:
    *   age and gender of patient
    *   position of patient
    *   patient's level of consciousness at scene
    *   location of injury
    *   presence or absence of exit wound
    *   type of weapon used
    *   treatment
    *   vital signs
    *   approximate amount of blood lost
    *   who removed clothing
    *   who received clothing (chain of evidence)
    *   who received the patient
    *   information provided by the patient

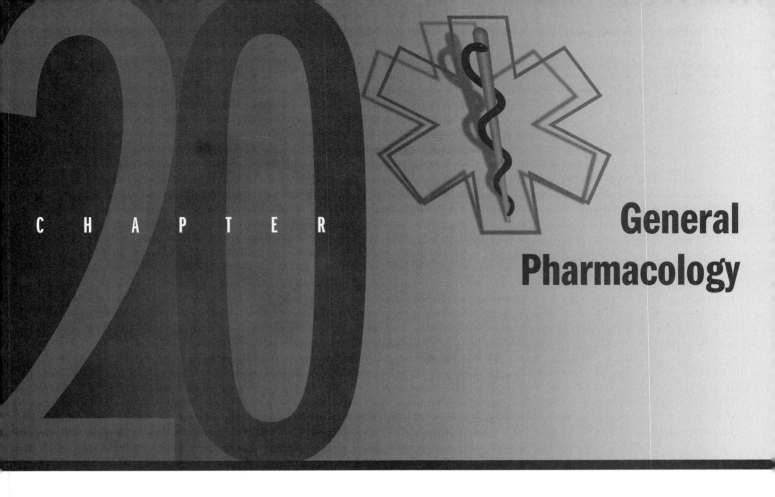

C H A P T E R

General Pharmacology

Reading Assignment: Chapter 20, pgs. 334–346

OBJECTIVES

1. Explain the rationale for administering medications.

2. Identify medications carried on the EMS vehicle by both generic and trade names.

3. Identify medications with which the EMT can assist the patient in administering by both generic and trade names.

4. Discuss the different forms that medications can be found in and the characteristics of different routes of administration.

5. Understand medication labels and assist the patient with self-administration of these medications.

INTRODUCTION

Healthcare providers use a variety of medications to treat their patients. Medications are chemicals that change the way the body functions. Pharmacology is the study of these medications. There is an extensive use of medications in emergency situations, primarily to treat the cause of the disease or to relieve symptoms of an underlying problem. Drugs can be beneficial but also can be dangerous if used incorrectly.

Actions, side effects, indications and contraindications are critical characteristics of each medication. This chapter discusses general pharmacology, including routes of administration and other considerations that the EMT must understand.

REVIEW QUESTIONS

Please circle one correct answer for each question.

1. Which of the following are useful effects of medications? (A 4-1.6)
    a. pain relief
    b. decreasing the work of the heart
    c. absorbing poisonous materials from the stomach
    d. all of the above

2. Medications that are usually carried on the basic EMS unit include all of the following **except**: (C 4-1.1 & 2)
    a. morphine
    b. activated charcoal
    c. oral glucose
    d. oxygen

3. The EMT-B, with approval by medical direction, may assist the patient in taking which of the following medications? (C 4-1.3, 4)
    a. morphine, lasix, and atenolol
    b. morphine, lanoxin, and atenolol
    c. inhaler, epinephrine, and nitroglycerin
    d. inhaler, atropine, and nitroglycerin

4. Each medication has several names. The two most important names for the EMT to know are: (C 4-1.2, 4)
    a. chemical name and the trade name
    b. generic name and the trade name
    c. generic name and the chemical name
    d. brand name and the chemical name

5. How many generic names can a drug have? (C 4-1.2, 4)
    a. 4
    b. 2
    c. 5
    d. 1

6. The generic name is a simple form of the complex chemical name. It is assigned by the government and is officially listed in a book called U.S. Pharmacopeia. (C 4-1.2, 4)
    a. true
    b. false

7. Which names are given to a drug by the companies that sell the drug? (P 4-1.8)

   a. trade name or brand name
   b. trade name or generic name
   c. trade name or chemical name
   d. brand name or generic name

8. Proventil and Ventolin are trade names of the same generic drug known as: (C 4-1.4)

   a. Albuterol
   b. Nuprin
   c. Primatene
   d. Acetaminophen

9. Tablets are made from: (C 4-1.5)

   a. a gel
   b. a liquid
   c. a compressed powder
   d. a gas

10. Nitroglycerin spray and tablets are given to the patient: (P 4-1.7)

   a. orally and swallowed
   b. sublingually
   c. intravenously
   d. transdermally

11. What form of drug is Oral Glucose? (C 4-1.5)

   a. gel
   b. suspension
   c. tablet
   d. injectable liquid

12. What form of drug is activated charcoal? (C 4-1.5)

   a. injectable liquid
   b. gas
   c. suspension
   d. gel

13. How is epinephrine administered to a patient via an automatic device? (P 4-1.8)

   a. SQ injection
   b. sublingually
   c. orally
   d. inhalation

14. The route of medication taken by mouth is known as: (A 4-1.6)

   a. PO
   b. SL
   c. IM
   d. SC

15. A drug given by subcutaneous injection is injected: (P 4-1.7)

   a. into the muscle
   b. into the tongue
   c. under the skin in the fat
   d. into a vein

16. Unconscious patients can safely be given medications by mouth. (A 4-1.7)

    a. true
    b. false

17. An EMT-B can assist a patient in taking medications by doing all of the following **except**: (A 4-1.7)

    a. finding the medication
    b. getting water for the patient
    c. helping identify the medication
    d. directly administering an intramuscular injection

18. An indication for assisting a patient to take nitroglycerin is: (A 4-1.7)

    a. headache
    b. chest pain
    c. asthma
    d. allergic reaction

19. A contraindication to nitroglycerin is: (A 4-1.7)

    a. high blood pressure
    b. low blood pressure
    c. headache
    d. chest pain

20. A patient must be thoroughly assessed both before and after a medication is given.

    a. true
    b. false

Scenario

Read each scenario. Write the answers to the corresponding questions in the space provided.

SCENARIO #1:

You and your partner have responded to a patient having difficulty breathing. The patient is a 17-year-old female and is in obvious respiratory distress. The patient states she has had similar problems before and that she uses an inhaler that is in the medicine cabinet. She states she did not use it today because her mother is out of town.

The patient's respiratory rate is 24 with expiratory wheezes. Her blood pressure is 120/80, and her pulse is 100. You retrieve the inhaler and note it is albuterol, but was prescribed for the patient's mother.

1. What should be done for this patient?

    _____

    _____

    _____

    _____

continued

2. Is it appropriate to administer the albuterol?

_____

_____

_____

_____

3. What should be done for the patient en route to the emergency department?

_____

_____

_____

_____

CHAPTER 20 ANSWERS TO REVIEW QUESTIONS

1. d	5. d	9. c	13. a	17. d
2. a	6. a	10. b	14. a	18. b
3. c	7. a	11. a	15. c	19. b
4. b	8. a	12. c	16. b	20. a

SCENARIO SOLUTIONS

Scenario #1

1. The patient should be placed on oxygen.
2. Since the albuterol is not prescribed for the patient, the EMT should not assist the patient in taking it.
3. Oxygen should be continued and the patient should be reassessed.

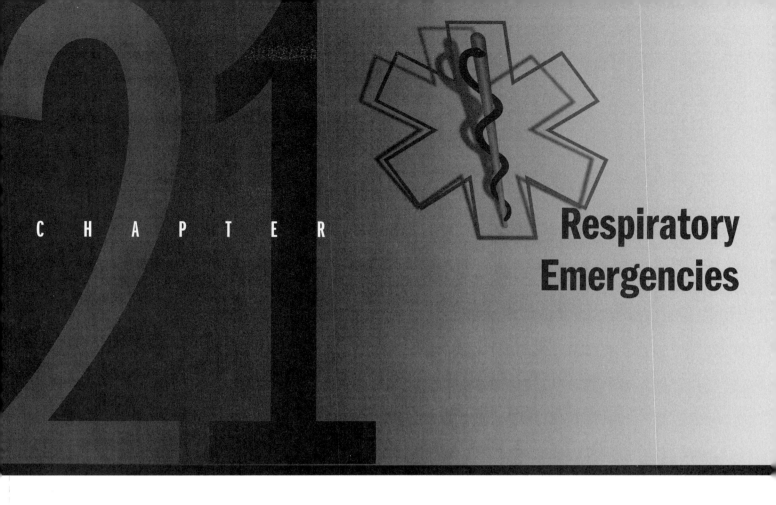

CHAPTER 21

Respiratory Emergencies

Reading Assignment: Chapter 21, pgs. 347–360

OBJECTIVES

1. Relate the physiology of the respiratory system to the signs and symptoms of inadequate breathing.

2. Describe the assessment and prehospital care of the patient who has breathing difficulty.

3. Describe the special considerations needed to care for infants and children with respiratory emergencies.

4. List the indications and contraindications for inhaler medications and demonstrate the steps required to assist with inhaler administration.

5. List the signs and symptoms of respiratory distress and demonstrate the ability to intervene appropriately with supplemental oxygen and/or airway management and artificial ventilation.

INTRODUCTION

A common chief complaint is shortness of breath. The EMT plays an important role in the management and transport of patients who have respiratory distress. Rapid assessment and prompt intervention in the prehospital setting can have a dramatic impact on patient outcome.

This chapter reviews the more common respiratory emergencies and discusses appropriate patient management. It discusses common respiratory disorders encountered in the field and focuses on important signs and symptoms that require intervention by the EMT. This chapter also covers oxygen therapy and the techniques for assisting with inhaler administration.

REVIEW QUESTIONS

Please circle one correct answer for each question.

1. The respiratory system serves two basic functions: (C 4-2.1)

   a. it supplies oxygen to the blood and removes carbon dioxide from the blood
   b. it supplies nitrogen to the blood and removes oxygen from the blood
   c. it supplies oxygen to the blood and removes carbon monoxide from the blood
   d. it supplies carbon monoxide to the blood and removes oxygen from the blood

2. A common byproduct produced by the cell's use of oxygen is: (C 4-2.1)

   a. carbon monoxide
   b. carbon dioxide
   c. sulfur dioxide
   d. carbon trioxide

3. The most common respiratory or breathing disorders the EMT will encounter in the field are: (C 4-2.2)

   a. COPD and hyperventilation
   b. pulmonary embolism and hemothorax
   c. COPD and asthma
   d. pulmonary embolism and hyperventilation

4. Signs and symptoms of respiratory distress related to COPD may include: (C 4-2.2)

   a. dyspnea
   b. productive cough
   c. agitation
   d. all of the above

5. Signs and symptoms of a severe asthma attack may include all of the following **except**: (4-2.1)

   a. no lung sounds and cardiac arrest
   b. respiratory arrest and irritability
   c. confusion and lethargy
   d. crepitus and abdominal distention

6. Chronic obstructive pulmonary disease is most often seen in: (4-2.2)

    a. infants that can't drink milk
    b. children that eat smoked meat
    c. older people with a history of smoking
    d. young adults that drink

7. Signs and symptoms of hyperventilation may include: (C 4-2.2)

    a. an increased respiratory rate
    b. tingling in the hands and feet
    c. agitation
    d. all of the above

8. A patient who appears to be hyperventilating should be: (C 4-2.3)

    a. instructed to increase the rate of respiration
    b. instructed to relax and slow their breathing
    c. be fitted with an oxygen mask without oxygen
    d. instructed to breathe into a small bag

9. Hyperventilation is always caused by anxiety. (C 4-2.2)

    a. true
    b. false

10. Pulmonary edema is a condition in which fluid accumulates in the airways. The most common cause of pulmonary edema is: (C 4-2.2)

    a. narcotic overdose
    b. bee stings
    c. congestive heart failure
    d. fluid overload

11. The signs and symptoms of pulmonary edema may include: (C 4-2.2)

    a. pink frothy sputum and distended neck veins
    b. dyspnea and hypoxia
    c. breath sounds with coarse crackles
    d. all of the above

12. Neck vein distention, secondary to pulmonary edema is caused by: (C 4-2.2)

    a. congestion in the heart and liver
    b. congestion in the heart and lungs
    c. congestion in the heart and kidneys
    d. congestion in the liver and lungs

13. Patients with pulmonary edema should be given high-flow oxygen and transported immediately. (C 4-2.3)

    a. true
    b. false

14. Croup is an infection that affects the upper airway and is caused by: (C 4-2.10)

    a. a virus
    b. bacteria
    c. parasites
    d. drugs

15. Croup is usually seen in what age group? (C 4-2.10)

    a. 1 month to 3 months
    b. 6 months to 3 years
    c. 3 years to 6 years
    d. 5 years to 8 years

16. Signs and symptoms of croup include all of the following **except**: (C 4-2.2)

    a. agitation
    b. "barking" cough
    c. low-grade fever
    d. drooling

17. Epiglottitis is an infection of the epiglottis caused by: (C 4-2.10)

    a. a parasite
    b. bacteria
    c. a virus
    d. drugs

18. Signs and symptoms of epiglottitis include: (C 4-2.2)

    a. a quiet child that sits still
    b. an excessive amount of saliva
    c. a high fever
    d. all of the above

19. Chronic bronchitis is a form of obstructive lung disease characterized by excess mucus production in the airways, causing cough and airway obstruction. (C 4-2.2)

    a. true
    b. false

20. Signs and symptoms of asthma include all of the following **except**: (C 4-2.2)

    a. dyspnea and difficulty exhaling
    b. wheezing and a dry cough
    c. an overexpanded chest
    d. bradycardia and jaundice

21. A pulmonary embolism causes hypoxia by: (C 4-2.1)

    a. blocking the aorta
    b. blocking the inferior vena cava
    c. blocking the carotid artery
    d. blocking a pulmonary artery

22. A pneumothorax is caused by: (C 4-2.1)

    a. air in the pleural space
    b. blood in the pleural space
    c. plasma in the pleural space
    d. water in the pleural space

23. A hemothorax is caused by: (C 4-2.1)

    a. air in the pleural space
    b. blood in the pleural space
    c. plasma in the heart space
    d. water in the abdomen

24. Signs and symptoms of a pneumothorax can include all of the following **except**: (C 4-2.2)

   a. dyspnea and chest pain
   b. fast respiratory rate and diminished breath sounds
   c. changes in LOC and cyanosis
   d. equal, bilateral breath sounds

25. Pneumonia may be caused by: (C 4-2.1)

   a. bacteria
   b. viruses
   c. fungi
   d. all of the above

26. Signs and symptoms of pneumonia include: (C 4-2.2)

   a. fever and chills
   b. productive cough
   c. dyspnea and hypoxia
   d. all of the above

27. Which of the following indications must be present before the EMT can assist with an inhaler: (C 4-2.4, 8)

   a. The patient exhibits signs and symptoms of respiratory distress.
   b. The patient has a currently prescribed hand held inhaler.
   c. The EMT has specific authorization by medical control to assist with inhalers.
   d. all of the above

28. Which of the following is important information about the patient with respiratory difficulties? (C 4-2.9)

   a. onset and duration of symptoms
   b. the presence of associated symptoms
   c. the patient's past medical history
   d. all of the above

29. Which of the following are normal respiratory rates: (C 4-2.1)

   a. adults 20–24/min; children 15–30/min; infants 25–50/min
   b. adults 8–24/min; children 15–30/min; infants 25–100/min
   c. adults 12–24/min; children 15–30/min; infants 25–50/min
   d. adults 8–30/min; children 15–30/min; infants 25–50/min

30. A patient with a head injury or drug overdose may have an irregular pattern of respirations. (C 4-2.2)

   a. true
   b. false

31. The quality of respirations is determined by: (C 4-2.7)

   a. listening to breath sounds
   b. watching for equal chest expansion
   c. assessing the effort required for breathing
   d. all of the above

32. Patients who are in acute respiratory distress are often unable to talk or may talk in one- to two-word sentences. (C 4-2.2)

   a. true
   b. false

33. A patient who has agonal respirations or is in respiratory arrest requires immediate: (C 4-2.5, 6)

    a. oxygen by mask
    b. artificial ventilation with 100% oxygen
    c. artificial ventilation with 40% oxygen
    d. oxygen via nasal cannula

34. An unresponsive patient with snoring or gurgling sounds during breathing indicates: (C 4-2.2)

    a. inadequate upper airway control
    b. a need for an artificial airway adjunct
    c. a need for suctioning
    d. all of the above

35. Inadequate breathing could be indicated by all of the following **except**: (C 4-2.7)

    a. the use of accessory muscles
    b. nasal flaring
    c. a patient sitting upright and leaning forward
    d. normal rise and fall of the chest wall

36. Which of the following are the most important interventions for a patient with inadequate breathing: (C 4-2.9)

    a. establish and maintain an adequate airway
    b. administer supplemental oxygen
    c. provide artificial ventilation when needed
    d. all of the above

37. Any patient with signs of hypoxia needs high-flow oxygen, regardless of a history of COPD. (C 4-2.5)

    a. true
    b. false

38. The EMT should let the nontrauma patient stay in whatever position is most comfortable, since this will decrease the patient's anxiety. (C 4-2.9)

    a. true
    b. false

39. The side effects of bronchodilators include: (C 4-2.8)

    a. increased pulse rate
    b. tremors
    c. nervousness and agitation
    d. all of the above

40. An alternative to oxygen administration by mask for children is the blow-by method. (C 4-2.9)

    a. true
    b. false

Scenario

Read each scenario. Write the answers to the corresponding questions in the space provided.

SCENARIO #1:

You are called to the scene where a 60-year-old male has suddenly become short of breath. Upon arrival you find a patient who appears anxious and quite short of breath. The patient is sitting bolt upright with his hands on his knees and arms straight.

The patient has a history of heavy smoking. The patient is conscious, alert, and his skin appears blue. He responds to questions with one- and two-word sentences and seems upset with your questions. The patient has very noisy respiratory sounds upon auscultation.

1. What signs and symptoms of respiratory distress are present in this patient?

_____

_____

_____

_____

2. What steps would you take to manage this patient effectively at the scene and during transport?

_____

_____

_____

_____

CHAPTER 21 ANSWERS TO REVIEW QUESTIONS

1. a	8. b	16. d	24. d	32. a
2. b	9. b	17. b	25. d	33. b
3. c	10. c	18. d	26. d	34. d
4. d	11. d	19. a	27. d	35. d
5. d	12. b	20. d	28. d	36. d
6. c	13. a	21. d	29. c	37. a
7. d	14. a	22. a	30. a	38. a
	15. b	23. b	31. d	39. d
				40. a

SCENARIO SOLUTIONS

Scenario #1

1. In this patient the signs and symptoms of respiratory distress are as follows:
- anxiety
- shortness of breath
- position of patient
- skin color
- unable to talk in more than two-word sentences
- noisy respiration

2. The following five steps should be taken to manage this patient effectively:
   a. high flow oxygen
   b. monitor vital signs
   c. rapid transport
   d. allow the patient to sit upright
   e. develop a detailed past medical history

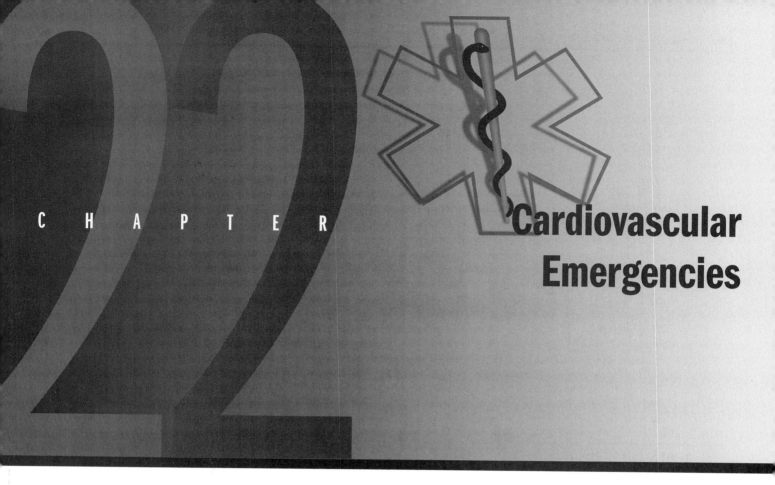

Cardiovascular Emergencies

Reading Assignment: Chapter 22, pgs. 361–384

OBJECTIVES

1. Describe the anatomy and function of the cardiovascular system.

2. Identify signs and symptoms of a cardiovascular problem and identify the necessary interventions for standard cardiac care.

3. Describe the emergency cardiac care system, including the rationale, indications, and contraindications for early defibrillation; the importance of early advanced cardiac life support (ACLS); the relationship between basic life support and ACLS providers; and the role of the EMT within this system.

4. Summarize the rationale for and operation of automated external defibrillators (AEDs), including:

   The various types of AEDs and their operating procedures.

   The rationale for and importance of routine AED maintenance using the operator's shift checklist or device-specific manufacturer's recommendations for maintenance.

   The assessment of patient response to defibrillation and the components of postresuscitation care.

   The steps required to manage persistent or recurrent ventricular fibrillation with and without the presence of ACLS providers.

5. Discuss the role of medical direction and continuing education with the use of AEDs, including the importance of case reviews.

6. Explain the rationale for facilitating the use of nitroglycerin for patients with chest pain, including the indications, contraindications, and side effects of the drug.

INTRODUCTION

Each year nearly 500,000 people in the United States die as a result of coronary artery disease. Half of these deaths occur outside the hospital. Sudden death is the first sign of cardiac disease in 50% of these out-of-hospital deaths.

This chapter discusses the anatomy and physiology of the cardiovascular system, and follows with a discussion of cardiovascular pathophysiology, including acute myocardial infarction (AMI) and congestive heart failure (CHF). It reviews assessment of the cardiac patient, rationale and components of standard cardiac care.

REVIEW QUESTIONS

Please circle one correct answer for each question.

1. How many chambers are in the heart? (C 4-3.1)

   a. 5
   b. 3
   c. 4
   d. 6

2. The two upper chambers of the heart are the: (C 4-3.1)

   a. ventricles
   b. atria
   c. aorta
   d. vena cava

3. The right half of the heart receives blood from the veins of the body, which empty into the right atrium through the superior and inferior vena cavae. (C 4-3.1)

   a. true
   b. false

4. The right ventricle pumps oxygen poor blood to the lungs through the: (C 4-3.1)

   a. pulmonary veins
   b. aorta
   c. vena cava
   d. pulmonary arteries

5. What happens to the blood as it passes through the pulmonary capillaries? (C 4-3.1)

    a. oxygen is added and carbon dioxide removed
    b. carbon dioxide is added and oxygen is removed
    c. oxygen is added and carbon dioxide is added
    d. oxygen is removed and carbon dioxide is removed

6. After receiving oxygen and eliminating carbon dioxide in the lungs, the blood enters the left atrium via: (C 4-3.1)

    a. the pulmonary veins
    b. the aorta
    c. the pulmonary arteries
    d. the vena cava

7. How many valves are in the heart? (C 4-3.1)

    a. 5
    b. 6
    c. 4
    d. 8

8. Where are the valves located in the heart? (C 4-3.1)

    a. two valves are located between the atria and ventricles
    b. one valve is located between the right ventricle and the pulmonary artery
    c. one valve is located between the left ventricle and the aorta
    d. all of the above

9. What is the normal order of the electrical conduction system of the heart? (C 4-3.1)

    a. atrioventricular (AV) node, sinoatrial (SA) node, ventricles
    b. ventricles, AV node, SA node
    c. SA node, ventricles, AV node
    d. SA node, AV node, ventricles

10. An abnormal rhythm of the heart is called a(n): (C 4-3.3)

    a. arrhythmia
    b. paranormal rhythm
    c. rhythmia
    d. pararhythm

11. Bradycardia usually refers to a heart rate of: (C 4-3.3)

    a. less than 70 BPM
    b. less than 60 BPM
    c. greater than 60 BPM
    d. less than 100 BPM

12. Tachycardia usually refers to a heart rate of: (C 4-3.3)

    a. greater than 100 BPM
    b. greater than 80 BPM
    c. less than 100 BPM
    d. less than 60 BPM

13. Ventricular fibrillation is an arrhythmia in that the entire heart is receiving random, disorganized, electrical impulses, whereby coordinated contraction cannot take place. (C 4-3.3)

    a. true
    b. false

14. Defibrillation is designed to temporarily halt the electrical activity of the heart, to allow the normal conduction system to regain control in the heart, enabling effective contraction. (C 4-3.3)

    a. true
    b. false

15. An arrhythmia that may require defibrillation is: (C 4-3.3)

    a. normal sinus rhythm
    b. pulseless ventricular tachycardia
    c. an agonal rhythm
    d. atrial fibrillation

16. Arteries are blood vessels that carry blood to the heart. (C 4-3.1)

    a. true
    b. false

17. The pulmonary arteries carry: (C 4-3.1)

    a. deoxygenated blood
    b. plasma only
    c. oxygen-rich blood
    d. oxygenated blood

18. The largest artery in the body is the: (C 4-3.1)

    a. femoral
    b. aorta
    c. carotid
    d. pulmonary

19. The heart is supplied with blood from the: (C 4-3.1)

    a. coronary arteries
    b. carotid arteries
    c. radial arteries
    d. pulmonary arteries

20. The smallest branches of the arteries are the: (C 4-3.1)

    a. venules
    b. veins
    c. vena cava
    d. arterioles

21. Capillaries surround the body's cells and supply them with oxygen and nutrients. (C 4-3.1)

    a. true
    b. false

22. Veins are vessels that carry blood: (C 4-3.1)

    a. to the legs
    b. toward the heart
    c. to the body
    d. to the lungs

23. The largest veins in the body are the: (C 4-3.1)

    a. ascending and descending aorta
    b. jugular veins
    c. superior and inferior vena cavae
    d. saphenous veins

24. Which blood cells contain hemoglobin and carry oxygen? (C 4-3.1)

    a. white blood cells
    b. plasma
    c. platelets
    d. red blood cells

25. In general, a systolic pressure of 120 mm Hg is needed to palpate a radial pulse, 60 mm Hg to palpate a carotid pulse, and 70 mm Hg to palpate a femoral pulse. (C 4-3.1)

    a. true
    b. false

26. Inadequate blood flow to a tissue is called: (C 4-3.8)

    a. anemia
    b. ischemia
    c. uremia
    d. hypertension

27. Angina pectoris is the term given to chest pain brought on by exercise and is usually: (C 4-3.8)

    a. relieved by rest
    b. not relieved by rest
    c. experienced when sleeping
    d. unrelated to exercise

28. A myocardial infarction may cause the irreversible death of part of the heart muscle. (C 4-3.1)

    a. true
    b. false

29. The most common signs of right heart failure are: (C 4-3.1)

    a. distended neck veins and swelling of the upper extremities
    b. flat neck veins and swelling of the upper extremities
    c. flat neck veins and swelling of the lower extremities
    d. distended neck veins and swelling in the lower extremities

30. Cardiogenic shock is a state of hypoperfusion caused by inadequate pumping action by the heart. (C 4-3.1)

    a. true
    b. false

31. If a patient complains of severe substernal chest pain and shortness of breath, the EMT should: (C 4-3.2)

    a. check the patient's blood pressure
    b. administer a high concentration of oxygen
    c. call medical control
    d. place the patient in a prone position

32. The typical findings with cardiac related chest pain include all of the following **except**: (C 4-3.2)

    a. pain originating in the center of the chest
    b. dull or squeezing in nature
    c. radiation down the left arm
    d. radiation down the right leg

33. Standard cardiac care for the EMT-B includes all of the following **except**: (C 4-3.2, 7)

    a. placing the patient in a position of comfort
    b. providing supplemental oxygen
    c. assisting with administration of the patient's nitroglycerin when indicated and authorized by medical control
    d. administration of lidocaine

34. Supplemental oxygen increases the content of oxygen in the blood, which helps deliver oxygen to areas of decreased blood flow. (C 4-3.8 and 9)

    a. true
    b. false

35. Nitroglycerin (NTG): (C 4-3.42)

    a. relaxes and dilates blood vessels
    b. dilates the coronary arteries
    c. can cause hypotension
    d. all of the above

36. Indications for NTG include: (C 4-3.41)

    a. chest pain
    b. a low blood pressure
    c. allergy to nitrates
    d. all of the above

37. Contraindications for NTG include: (C 4-3.42)

    a. systolic blood pressure less than 120 mm Hg
    b. head injury
    c. the patient has taken two NTG tablets already
    d. the patient has taken five NTG tablets already

38. The dosage of NTG is one tablet (or one to two puffs of NTG spray), administered sublingually (under the tongue) every 3–5 minutes until pain is relieved, up to a maximum of: (A 4-3.46)

    a. 3 doses
    b. 6 doses
    c. 4 doses
    d. 5 doses

39. The EMT may assist a patient in taking his or her nitroglycerin when the patient has a current prescription and has chest pain consistent with angina: (C 4-3.12, 41)

    a. without contacting medical control
    b. with your partner's approval
    c. with authorization from medical control
    d. with the policeman's approval

40. The most common initial rhythm in cardiac arrest is VF and:
(C 4-3.3)

    a. the definitive treatment for VF is defibrillation
    b. the likelihood of successful defibrillation diminishes rapidly
       after onset of VF
    c. normal sinus rhythm
    d. a and b

41. Early defibrillation by non-ACLS personnel has been shown to
decrease the urgency for other ACLS interventions, such as: (C 4-3.3)

    a. endotracheal intubation
    b. IV line placement
    c. drug administration
    d. all of the above

42. The four links in the chain of survival are: (C 4-3.5)

    a. early access, early CPR, early defibrillation, early ACLS
    b. early access, early CPR, early defibrillation, early surgery
    c. early access, early CPR, early reporting, early ACLS
    d. early access, early CPR, early defibrillation, better response times

43. Prompt and effective CPR allows time for interventions such as
defibrillation and ACLS measures to be effective. (C 4-3.30)

    a. true
    b. false

44. Proper AED operation depends on: (C 4-3.25)

    a. a thorough knowledge of established protocols
    b. frequent practice with the device
    c. routine defibrillator and battery maintenance
    d. all of the above

45. A fully automated defibrillator delivers shocks to the patient
without any action by the EMT except turning the power on and
applying the electrodes. (C 4-3.15, 16)

    a. true
    b. false

46. A semi-automated defibrillator instructs the EMT to deliver shocks.
(C 4-3.15, 16)

    a. true
    b. false

47. Common mistakes that occur with the use of an AED include:
(C 4-3.17, 19)

    a. incorrect application of electrodes
    b. failure to deliver a shock when the device indicates one
    c. not knowing how to operate the device
    d. all of the above

48. One of the most common causes of AED malfunction is: (C 4-3.39)

    a. electrode placement
    b. moving vehicle
    c. battery failure
    d. operator error

49. Automated external defribillator checklists should be used daily to ensure proper function. (C 4-3.34)

   a. true
   b. false

50. With defibrillator maintenance, regular tests and frequent practice, errors in AED use can be minimized. (C 4-3.34, 43)

   a. true
   b. false

51. How quickly can an AED deliver a shock after the EMT is at the patient's side? (C 4-3.22)

   a. within 1 minute
   b. 3 minutes
   c. 5 minutes
   d. 4 minutes

52. Advantages of automated external defibrillators include: (C 4-3.21)

   a. shocks with "hands off" electrodes
   b. more surface area for defibrillation
   c. reliability
   d. all of the above

53. Unless ALS personnel are on scene or a variance is permitted by local medical control, the patient should be transported when which of the following occurs: (C 4-3.26, 27)

   a. the patient regains a pulse
   b. six shocks are delivered
   c. three consecutive no shock messages are given separated by one minute of CPR
   d. all of the above

54. The most common cause of cardiac arrest in children is: (C 4-3.6)

   a. cardiac failure
   b. brain abnormalities
   c. respiratory compromise
   d. fright

55. Due to artifact produced by a moving ambulance, the AED cannot accurately analyze while the vehicle is moving. (C 4-3.24)

   a. true
   b. false

56. When pulselessness and apnea are confirmed: (C 4-3.18)

   a. CPR is resumed by a partner while the AED is attached to the patient
   b. IVs are started by the basic EMT
   c. AEDs should not be used
   d. AEDS are of no use

57. Automated external defibrillator electrodes are positioned below the clavicle just to the left of the upper part of the sternum and over the lower ribs on the left side of the chest wall. (C 4-3.23)

   a. true
   b. false

58. Pulse checks should not be performed between stacked shocks because they: (C 4-3.29)

 a. increase the risk to the EMT
 b. are not reliable
 c. lengthen the time needed for defibrillation
 d. all of the above

59. Defibrillation is more important than CPR when VF or pulseless VT is present. (C 4-3.11)

 a. true
 b. false

60. Post-resuscitation care components include: (C 4-3.32)

 a. breathing assessment
 b. pulse assessment
 c. oxygen administration
 d. all of the above

61. Automated external defibrillator operation by EMTs can only take place under the authority of local medical control and each case in that an AED is used should be reviewed by the local medical director. (C 4-3.40)

 a. true
 b. false

62. Documented use of the AED for case reviews should include written reports, voice-electrocardiogram (ECG) tape recordings, and digitized ECG. (C 4-3.38)

 a. true
 b. false

Scenario

Read each scenario. Write the answers to the corresponding questions in the space provided.

SCENARIO #1:
You are called to the scene where a 55-year-old male has been complaining of weakness and difficulty breathing. When you and your partner approach the patient he is supine on the floor. The son, who is on the scene, states he caught his father just before he fell. He believes that his father has stopped breathing.

 The patient is not breathing and has no pulse. You are 15 minutes away from the nearest ALS unit.

1. What steps should be taken to manage this patient?

_____

_____

_____

_____

CHAPTER 22 ANSWERS TO REVIEW QUESTIONS

1. c	**14.** a	**27.** a	**40.** d	**53.** d
2. b	**15.** b	**28.** a	**41.** d	**54.** c
3. a	**16.** b	**29.** d	**42.** a	**55.** a
4. d	**17.** a	**30.** a	**43.** a	**56.** a
5. a	**18.** b	**31.** b	**44.** d	**57.** b
6. a	**19.** a	**32.** d	**45.** a	**58.** c
7. c	**20.** d	**33.** d	**46.** a	**59.** a
8. d	**21.** a	**34.** a	**47.** d	**60.** d
9. d	**22.** b	**35.** d	**48.** c	**61.** a
10. a	**23.** c	**36.** a	**49.** a	**62.** a
11. b	**24.** d	**37.** b	**50.** a	
12. a	**25.** b	**38.** a	**51.** a	
13. a	**26.** b	**39.** c	**52.** d	

SCENARIO SOLUTIONS

Scenario #1:

1. To manage this patient, the following steps should be taken:
   a. confirm cardiac arrest
   b. start CPR
   c. attach AED
   d. stop CPR
   e. perform an analysis of the cardiac rhythm
   f. deliver sets of three shocks as indicated
   g. call for an ALS unit
   h. have the son locate the patient's medications
   i. CPR is performed for one minute between sets of three shocks and any time a "no shock indicated" message is given and there is no pulse
   j. place airway adjuncts and ventilate with 100% oxygen coordination of patient care after ALS arrival place patient on backboard

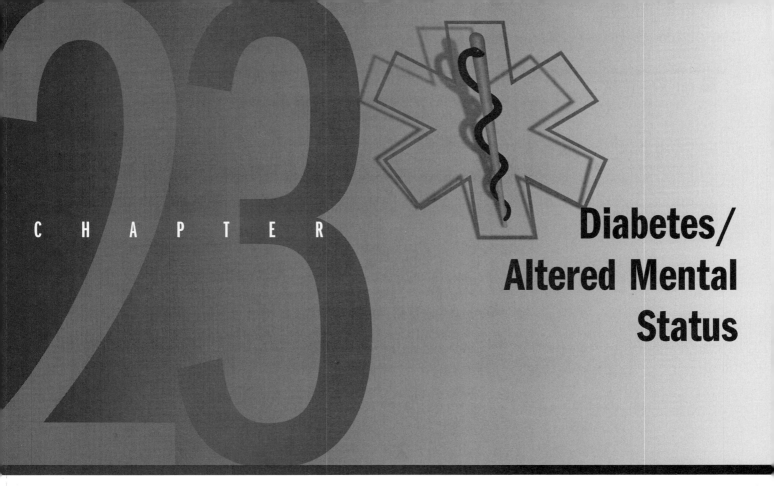

Diabetes/ Altered Mental Status

C H A P T E R 23

Reading Assignment: Chapter 23, pgs. 385–395

OBJECTIVES

1. Describe the evaluation and management of a patient who has a history of diabetes and has an altered mental status.

2. State the steps in the emergency medical care of a patient on diabetic medicine or with a history of diabetes who has an altered level of consciousness.

3. Identify the trade and generic names, forms, dosage, route of administration, and contraindications for oral glucose.

4. Describe a situation when medical direction or ALS intervention may be useful.

5. Describe the rationale for using glucose in a patient with altered mental status.

6. Demonstrate the steps in administration of oral glucose.

7. Demonstrate the assessment and documentation of patient response to oral glucose.

INTRODUCTION

Diabetes is a disease that affects more than 10 million Americans. Diabetic patients can present with emergencies related to either high or low blood sugar. This chapter discusses blood glucose levels and the field treatment of the diabetic patient.

REVIEW QUESTIONS

Please circle one correct answer for each question.

1. What substances are used by all cells of the body to produce energy?

   a. oxygen and carbon dioxide
   b. sugar and oxygen
   c. hemoglobin and nitrogen
   d. sugar and carbon dioxide

2. The hormone insulin facilitates: (C 4-4.4)

   a. the transmission of glucose from the blood stream into the cell
   b. the transmission of glucose from the cell into the blood stream
   c. the excretion of glucose from the cell
   d. the metabolization of ketones for energy

3. Insulin is made in special cells called beta cells that are found in the: (C 4-4.4)

   a. stomach
   b. liver
   c. pancreas
   d. spleen

4. Type I diabetics: (C 4-4.1)

   a. usually require insulin treatment and usually have adolescent onset
   b. do not require insulin treatment and usually start in late adulthood
   c. do not have signs and symptoms of diabetes
   d. produce too much insulin and must eat often

5. Type II diabetes is: (C 4-4.1)

   a. very rare except for newborn infants
   b. common in early adulthood and often associated with smoking
   c. common in slim adolescents
   d. more common in older patients and often associated with obesity

6. Which of the following is not a classic symptom of diabetes? (C 4-4.1)

   a. polyuria (increased urination)
   b. polyphagia (increased hunger and calorie intake)
   c. polydipsia (increased thirst)
   d. polyarthritis (inflammation of many joints)

7. Which of the following signs of diabetes can be attributed to the effects of low insulin levels? (C 4-4.1)

   a. increased blood glucose levels
   b. decreased fat use
   c. decreased protein use
   d. increased protein in the urine

8. Oral hypoglycemics are drugs that act to: (A 4-4.6)

   a. reduce glucose levels by increasing calorie intake
   b. decrease insulin production and increase glucose levels
   c. stimulate insulin release from the pancreas and increase the effectiveness of the existing insulin
   d. stimulate the use of fats and increase ketones

9. Which of the following are common oral hypoglycemics? (C 4-4.4)

   a. Micronase, DiaBeta, Glucotrol, Tolinase, and Diabinase
   b. Micronase, insulin, glucagon, Tolinase, and Diabinase
   c. insulin, DiaBeta, Glucotrol, Tolinase, and Diabinase
   d. Micro K, DiaBeta, Glucotrol, Tolinase, and Humulin

10. Which of the following are sources for insulin? (C 4-4.4)

    a. pork pancreas
    b. beef pancreas
    c. genetic engineering
    d. all of the above

11. Diabetic ketoacidosis (DKA) may be caused by: (C 4-4.1)

    a. a lack of adequate insulin
    b. an infection
    c. significant stress
    d. all of the above

12. In DKA the cells are not able to metabolize glucose, therefore the body begins to metabolize fats and proteins to provide an energy source for the cells. (C 4-4.1)

    a. true
    b. false

13. The DKA patient may present with which of the following signs and symptoms? (C 4-4.2)

    a. a fruity odor on the breath
    b. diuresis and dehydration
    c. change in level of consciousness
    d. all of the above

14. Which of the following are true concerning non-ketotic, hyperosmolar state (NKHS)? (C 4-4.1)

    a. fat and protein breakdown does not occur to the extent of DKA
    b. the patient will present with altered mental status
    c. the patient has extreme hyperglycemia
    d. all of the above

15. Hypoglycemia is: (C 4-4.3)

    a. high blood sugar
    b. low blood sugar
    c. high calorie intake
    d. low calorie use

16. Low blood sugar can cause: (C 4-4.3)

    a. altered levels of consciousness
    b. seizures
    c. brain damage
    d. all of the above

17. All of the following are clues that a patient may be a diabetic **except**: (C 4-4.1, 2)

    a. insulin bottles in the refrigerator
    b. needle marks on the thigh
    c. medic alert bracelets
    d. the presence of nitro patches on the chest

18. Pertinent questions to ask a diabetic patient include which of the following? (C 4-4.3)

    a. increased thirst, appetite, and urination
    b. medications, medication dose
    c. past episodes of diabetic complications, last meal
    d. all of the above

19. Diabetic patients with altered mental status may have impaired protective reflexes and require a jaw thrust, suctioning, nasal airway, or other airway maneuver. (C 4-4.2)

    a. true
    b. false

20. Kussmaul respiration characteristics are: (C 4-4.1)

    a. slow, deep breathing
    b. rapid, deep breathing
    c. shallow, agonal breathing
    d. rapid, shallow breathing

21. Which of the following is not a finding of the severely ill diabetic? (C 4-4.2)

    a. conscious and alert
    b. restlessness and confusion
    c. combativeness
    d. seizures or coma

22. Diabetic patients who are not effectively swallowing their saliva (drooling) should generally not be given oral glucose. (C 4-4.4)

    a. true
    b. false

23. Since, besides diabetes, many other reasons for altered mental states exist, medical direction should be sought when dealing with a patient that has a change in LOC. (C 4-4.5)

    a. true
    b. false

Scenario

Read each scenario. Write the answers to the corresponding questions in the space provided.

SCENARIO #1:

You and your partner respond to a residence where you find a 28-year-old female patient who is lying on the floor in the bedroom. The patient's husband informs you that the patient has a 15-year history of diabetes. You note that the patient is wearing a Medic-Alert bracelet. She has been feeling bad for the past two days, but has refused to see a physician.

This morning while preparing breakfast, the patient stated that she was "feeling shaky" and was going to lie down for a few minutes. When her husband went into the bedroom to check on her, he found her slumped against the bed. He immediately phoned 911.

Upon initial assessment, you find that the patient is pale, cool, and has clammy skin. She responds to verbal stimuli.

1. List three pertinent questions that you should ask the patient, her husband, or both.

_____

_____

_____

_____

2. What assessment and management steps should be taken for this patient?

_____

_____

_____

_____

CHAPTER 23 ANSWERS TO REVIEW QUESTIONS

1. b	6. d	11. d	16. d	21. a
2. a	7. a	12. a	17. d	22. a
3. c	8. c	13. d	18. d	23. a
4. a	9. a	14. d	19. a	
5. d	10. d	15. b	20. b	

SCENARIO SOLUTIONS

Scenario #1

1. The following are pertinent questions you should ask:
    - Has the patient eaten today?
    - Has the patient taken her insulin?
    - Has the patient had any illness?
    - Has the patient been eating more than usual?
    - Has the patient been drinking water more than usual?
    - Has the patient been urinating more than usual?

2. The following are steps that should be taken:
    a. Place the patient on high flow oxygen.
    b. Give the patient oral glucose based on medical control directives.
    c. Perform a thorough assessment and transport.
    d. Check for a Medic-Alert bracelet/necklace.

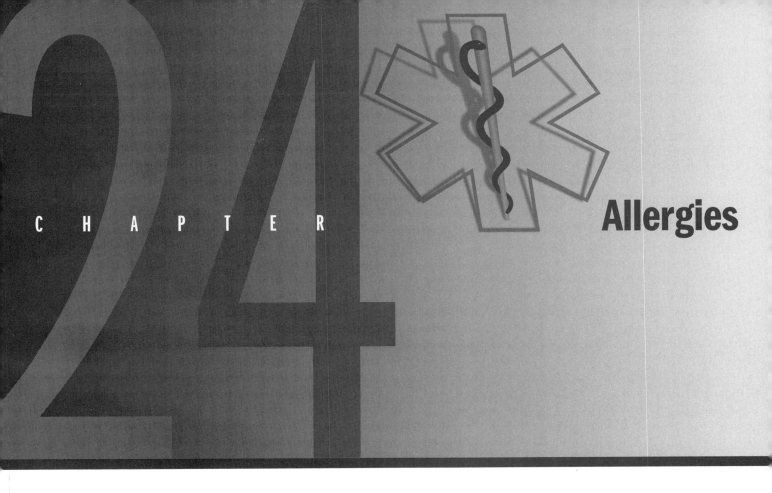

CHAPTER 24

Allergies

Reading Assignment: Chapter 24, pgs. 396–404

OBJECTIVES

1. Define allergic reaction.

2. Describe and identify urticaria.

3. Distinguish an anaphylactic reaction from a simple allergic reaction.

4. List the most common antigens to cause anaphylaxis.

5. List the indications for assisting a patient with the administration of epinephrine.

6. Describe the use of an epinephrine auto-injector.

7. Describe the use of a syringe to administer epinephrine.

INTRODUCTION

Allergic reactions are a response of the body's immune system when challenged by foreign substances. Allergic reactions range from a minor single system reaction to a life-threatening anaphylactic reaction.

Severe allergic reactions frequently cause death to occur within minutes of onset. This chapter discusses the proper assessment and management in the prehospital setting of the patient suffering from an allergic reaction.

REVIEW QUESTIONS

Please circle one correct answer for each question.

1. Antibodies are produced by the body to: (C 4-5.4)
   a. destroy antigens
   b. create antigens
   c. create antibiotics
   d. destroy antibiotics

2. The most common type of allergic reaction that requires transport to the hospital is a(n): (C 4-5.2)
   a. chronic hypersensitivity reaction
   b. immediate hypersensitivity reaction
   c. latent hyposensitivity reaction
   d. immediate hyposensitivity reaction

3. Which of the following are common types of antigens associated with an immediate hypersensitivity reaction: (C 4-5.4)
   a. insect venom, antibiotics
   b. injected penicillin, nuts
   c. shellfish, strawberries
   d. all of the above

4. Hypersensitivity reactions cause the release of what chemical from white blood cells? (C 4-5.4)
   a. antihistamine
   b. histamine
   c. hemoglobin
   d. glucose

5. What effects are due to the release of histamine? (C 4-5.1)
   a. vasodilation, leaking blood vessels
   b. vasoconstriction, leaking blood vessels
   c. vasoconstriction, high blood pressure
   d. vasoconstriction, vomiting

6. Vasodilation of the peripheral blood vessels causes: (C 4-5.4)
   a. hives
   b. urticaria
   c. a rash
   d. all of the above

7. Hives are characterized by: (C 4-5.1)
   a. raised, blanched, irregularly shaped lesions
   b. redness
   c. severe itching
   d. all of the above

8. Generalized vasodilation may lead to hypotension and shock. (P 4-5.9)

   a. true
   b. false

9. Histamine can cause all of the following **except**: (C 4-5.1)

   a. bronchodilation and wheezing
   b. watery eyes and a runny nose
   c. hives and vomiting
   d. difficulty breathing and shock

10. Which of the following are signs and symptoms of an anaphylactic reaction? (C 4-5.3)

    a. difficulty breathing
    b. shock
    c. rapid deterioration
    d. all of the above

11. What percentage of anaphylaxis patients die from shock and what percentage die from respiratory problems? (C 4-5.3)

    a. shock - 45%, respiratory - 55%
    b. shock - 55%, respiratory - 45%
    c. shock - 25%, respiratory - 75%
    d. shock - 5%, respiratory - 95%

12. Which of the following information would be important concerning an anaphylactic patient? (C 4-5.2)

    a. history of reaction, substance exposed to
    b. mode of exposure, effects, interventions
    c. progression of the effects, time period
    d. all of the above

13. What is the most dangerous complication of a severe allergic reaction? (C 4-5.2, 3)

    a. high blood pressure
    b. slow pulse rate
    c. kidney failure
    d. respiratory distress

14. Swelling of the tissues of the oropharynx and larynx can lead to airway obstruction, which will be evident by the presence of stridor. (C 4-5.2, 3)

    a. true
    b. false

15. Which of the following would be the best warning signs to indicate swollen vocal cords? (C 4-5.2, 3)

    a. swelling in the mouth or tongue
    b. swollen hands
    c. swollen abdomen
    d. swollen ankles

16. What causes wheezing in the lungs with the anaphylactic patient? (C 4-5.3)

    a. swelling and spasm of the tongue
    b. swelling and spasm of the smaller airway passages
    c. swelling and spasm of the large airway passages
    d. swelling and spasm of the pharynx

17. Which of the following are indications to assist a patient in administering his or her epinephrine? (C 4-5.7 and A 4-5.9)

    a. shock
    b. respiratory difficulty
    c. rapidly progressing symptoms
    d. all of the above

18. If a patient has a severe allergic reaction and does not have epinephrine, what should the EMT do? (C 4-5.6)

    a. early rapid transport
    b. complete assessment en route
    c. call medical control during transport of the patient
    d. all of the above

19. The management of allergic reactions is aimed at reducing further histamine release, and managing those problems that are already present. (C 4-5.2)

    a. true
    b. false

20. Early endotracheal intubation should be a consideration for the anaphylactic patient because: (C 4-5.4)

    a. all allergic reactions should be controlled with ET intubation
    b. the EOA is effective in most allergic reactions
    c. the ET should be placed while the patient is conscious
    d. increasing laryngeal edema may make it more difficult to accomplish later

21. What are the effects of epinephrine? (C 4-5.5)

    a. potent vasodilation and bronchodilation
    b. potent vasoconstriction and bronchodilation
    c. potent vasodilation and bronchoconstriction
    d. potent vasoconstriction and bronchoconstriction

22. Which of the following is not a side effect of epinephrine? (C 4-5.5)

    a. bradycardia
    b. angina
    c. hypertension
    d. myocardial ischemia

23. Epinephrine is safe for administration for minor allergic reactions in patients over 50 years of age. (C 4-5.5)

    a. true
    b. false

24. Which of the following packages of epinephrine contains a vial of epinephrine and a syringe that must be drawn up and injected? (C 4-5.5)

    a. Auto-jet
    b. Epi-Pen
    c. Ana-Kit
    d. Epi-Kit

25. What is the preloaded dose of epinephrine in the Epi-Pen? (C 4-5.5)

    a. 0.3 mg
    b. 3.0 mg
    c. 0.5 mg
    d. 1.0 mg

26. Epinephrine is administered in which layer of tissue from the Ana-Kit? (C 4-5.5)

    a. extradermal
    b. subcutaneous
    c. intravenous
    d. intramuscular

27. What should be done for the anaphylactic patient if no IV or medication is available? (C 4-5.5, 2)

    a. give the patient fluid by mouth
    b. no intervention is necessary
    c. transport in the shock position with supplemental oxygen
    d. none of the above

28. What is the primary drug treatment for anaphylaxis? (C 4-5.5 and 2)

    a. norepinephrine
    b. epinephrine
    c. diphenhydramine
    d. glucose

29. Which of the following is an auto-injector form of epinephrine? (C 4-5.5)

    a. Auto-jet
    b. Epi-Pen
    c. Ana-Kit
    d. Epi-Kit

Scenario

Read each scenario. Write the answers to the corresponding questions in the space provided.

SCENARIO #1:

You and your crew are at the station surveying your PCRs from this busy day. Suddenly a man walks into the station and, through audible wheezes, begs you to help him. You note instantly that this patient is in distress and begin to assess him as your partner retrieves the ambulance cot.

continued

Upon initial assessment, you note that the patient's face is displaying a bright red, flushed appearance. There is considerable edema around the neck and face. The patient exhibits signs and symptoms of rapidly progressing shock. His B/P begins to drop and his heart rate is tachycardic at a rate of 140.

About this time, the patient's wife comes running into the station and informs you that they were attending a Fourth of July picnic when her husband became ill. It seems that, approximately 8 years ago, the exact same thing had happened to him. At that time, the doctor determined that he was allergic to beef and advised him that he should not attempt to eat beef again. Unknown to the patient, the dinner casserole at the picnic consisted of beef and chicken!

1. What is the patient's immediate problem?

2. What is the probable cause of this patient's symptoms?

3. How would you manage his care?

CHAPTER 24 ANSWERS TO REVIEW QUESTIONS

1. a	7. d	13. d	19. a	25. a
2. b	8. a	14. a	20. d	26. b
3. d	9. a	15. a	21. b	27. c
4. b	10. d	16. b	22. a	28. b
5. a	11. c	17. d	23. b	29. b
6. d	12. d	18. d	24. c	

SCENARIO SOLUTIONS

Scenario #1:

1. You recognize the signs and symptoms as consistent with a severe anaphylactic reaction.

2. The patient's airway is compromised by swelling of the laryngeal tissue, causing wheezes. The patient is progressing into shock. Additional signs of shock include hypotension and tachycardia.

3. You should place the patient supine with legs elevated and attempt to maximize the airway patency. You assist ventilations with a BVM and 100% O$_2$.

Medical control directs you to administer an Epinephrine auto-injector and to transport the patient to the hospital immediately.

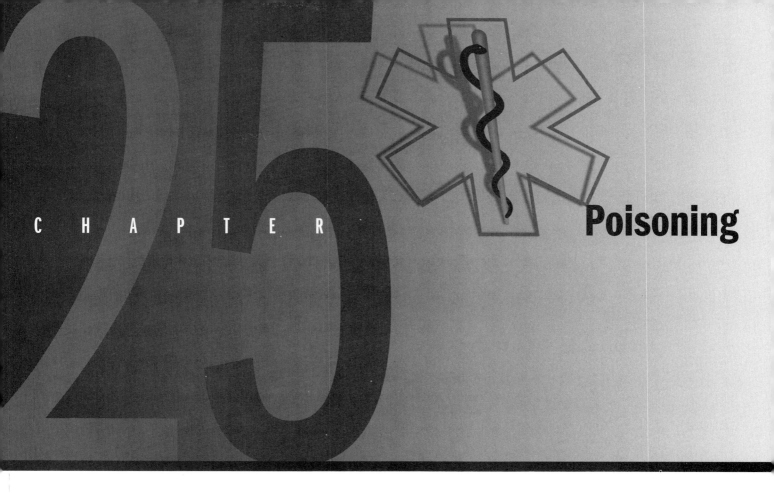

CHAPTER 25

Poisoning

Reading Assignment: Chapter 25, pgs. 405–417

OBJECTIVES

1. Define poison.
2. Describe the appropriate interaction with the poison control center.
3. Explain the various effects of poisons on the body.
4. List the forms of activated charcoal that are available.
5. Identify the appropriate circumstances to use ipecac and activated charcoal.
6. List the contraindications for activated charcoal.

INTRODUCTION

This chapter deals with those emergency situations caused by accidental or intentional poisonings. Poisoning is defined as the adverse effects of plants, foods, chemicals, or pharmaceutical agents on the body. Approximately 2.5 million human poison exposures were reported to poison control centers in 1993.

The majority of poison cases do not require long-term hospitalization. Prehospital care of poisoning patients is directed at assessment and stabilization of the airway, breathing, and circulation and may involve initiating decontamination in an attempt to reduce the poison concentration present at the scene.

REVIEW QUESTIONS

Please circle one correct answer for each question.

1. Poisoning may be defined as the beneficial effect of plants, food, chemicals, or drugs on the body. (C 4-6.2)

   a. true
   b. false

2. Poisoning can occur by: (C 4-6.1)

   a. inhalation
   b. absorption
   c. ingestion
   d. all of the above

3. Poison control centers are a primary resource for all of the following **except**: (C 4-6.4)

   a. information regarding toxicity
   b. information regarding management of poisoning
   c. information regarding STD transmission
   d. giving instructions regarding treatment of poisons

4. In cases of ingestion, medical control may recommend the use of activated charcoal to bind the poison in the intestine to prevent absorption into the bloodstream. (C 4-6.6)

   a. true
   b. false

5. The most commonly used medication to cause vomiting is: (Chapter 25, obj. 6)

   a. syrup of ipecac
   b. Benadryl
   c. activated charcoal
   d. Dramamine

6. Activated charcoal is used in all poisonings. (C 4-6.6)

   a. true
   b. false

7. Peak age incidence of poisoning include all of the following **except**:

   a. toddlers
   b. school age children
   c. adolescents
   d. kindergarten age children

8. The greatest risk to the patient who has had a narcotic overdose is: (C 4-6.5)

   a. addiction
   b. respiratory arrest
   c. cardiac arrest
   d. dependence

9. A few poisons have specific _____ that reverse or block the effect of the poison. (C 4-6.4)

   a. benefits
   b. detriments
   c. antidotes
   d. antibodies

10. The most common poisons in the 2-year-old age group include: (C 4-6.2)

   a. Duraspan and Spectracide
   b. household cleaning agents and medications
   c. gasoline and kerosene
   d. ammonium nitrate and diesel fuel

11. A centralized facility with access to poison information and toxicological consultation is called a:

   a. definitive care facility
   b. convalescence care facility
   c. Poison Control Center
   d. Communication Center

12. Poisoning by ingestion occurs when a poison is taken into the patient's: (C 4-6.1)

   a. mouth
   b. ear
   c. veins
   d. skin

13. Most absorption from ingested poisons takes place in the: (A 4-6.8)

   a. small intestine
   b. upper stomach
   c. large intestine
   d. descending colon

14. Some poisons are irritating or corrosive to the tissue that lines the mouth and esophagus. A person who ingests one of these poisons may experience: (C 4-6.2)

   a. burning
   b. swelling of the soft tissues of the mouth
   c. discomfort
   d. all of the above

15. If the concentration of the poisoning agent is high or exposure is prolonged, your primary concern as the attending EMT would be: (C 4-6.5)

   a. potential compromise to the upper airway
   b. pain/discomfort
   c. altered level of consciousness
   d. restlessness and anxiety

16. Recovering material that is still in the stomach, before it moves into the small intestine will reduce the amount absorbed. Methods used to counter poisonous material include: (C 4-6.6)

    a. syrup of ipecac
    b. gastric lavage ("pumping the stomach")
    c. administration of activated charcoal
    d. all of the above

17. In the course of handling a patient who was contaminated with dry lime, the skin of the responder, if not protected by appropriate personal protective gear, may become contaminated. Most of the time, adherence to the use of vinyl or latex gloves will provide adequate protection to the EMT. (P 4-6.11)

    a. true
    b. false

18. Rescuer safety is a significant issue in inhalation poisoning, because of all the following **except**: (C 4-6.4)

    a. the cause of the poisoning is not always obvious
    b. the EMT can be injured if self-contained breathing apparatus is not worn
    c. poisonous gas may be present
    d. the EMT is in no danger as long as no flames are visible

19. Management of poisoning is primarily supportive. Appropriate assessment of the poisoned patient includes all the following **except**: (P 4-6.11)

    a. airway, breathing, and circulation
    b. assessment of the level of consciousness
    c. assessment of adequacy of the gag reflex
    d. assessment of range of motion

20. Narcotic overdose depresses respirations and mental status, which can lead to compromise of the airway. A specific antidote for narcotic overdose is called _____. (C 4-6.3)

    a. syrup of ipecac
    b. activated charcoal
    c. Narcan (naloxone)
    d. Adenosine

21. In the prehospital field, thorough assessments of poisoned patients are necessary for medical control, poison control, or both, to determine whether field intervention is appropriate. (C 4-6.7)

    a. true
    b. false

22. If a container or material that contained the poison is present at the scene and can be safely transported, it is helpful to bring it with the patient because: (A 4-6.9)

    a. the quantity of material is important information
    b. emergency physicians may do a pill count on bottles of medication to estimate the number of pills ingested
    c. hospital staff may anticipate a higher risk to the patient and undertake more aggressive treatment if they have more specific information
    d. all of the above are true

23. Since the variety of poisons is wide, signs and symptoms can vary tremendously. Central nervous system symptoms may include all of the following **except**: (C 4-6.2)

    a. dizziness
    b. headache
    c. altered mental status
    d. abdominal pain

24. An order for activated charcoal administration must be obtained either online or offline. Accepted dosing is: (C 4-6.6)

    a. usually 0.5–1 g/kg of body weight
    b. usual adult dose of 15–30 g
    c. pediatric doses of 1.5–2 g
    d. pediatric doses of 10–15 g

25. Poisoning by injection includes: (C 4-6.1)

    a. substance abuse and envenomation by animals
    b. carbon monoxide and nitrogen
    c. carbon dioxide and ammonia
    d. lime and organophosphate powder

Scenario

Read each scenario. Write the answers to the corresponding questions in the space provided.

SCENARIO #1:

You and your EMT crew are responding to a call for assistance at a farmhouse where an elderly woman is lying in the yard. On arrival you are met by her frantic husband who explains that he has been spraying his garden for bugs. His wife came out to pick a few fresh tomatoes, unaware that her husband had just sprayed.

She exhibits a slow, bounding pulse rate and pinpoint pupils. Her respiratory rate is noted to be 12 breaths/min. She responds to verbal stimuli.

1. What do you expect to be the cause of the woman's condition?

_____

_____

_____

_____

continued

2. List your immediate treatment priorities.

_____

_____

_____

_____

3. Explain the need for medical direction in this scenario.

_____

_____

_____

_____

CHAPTER 25 ANSWERS TO REVIEW QUESTIONS

1.	b	**6.**	b	**11.**	c	**16.**	d	**21.**	b
2.	d	**7.**	c	**12.**	a	**17.**	b	**22.**	d
3.	c	**8.**	b	**13.**	a	**18.**	d	**23.**	d
4.	a	**9.**	c	**14.**	d	**19.**	d	**24.**	a
5.	a	**10.**	b	**15.**	a	**20.**	c	**25.**	a

SCENARIO SOLUTIONS

Scenario #1:

1. Suspect contact poisoning, possibly organophosphate poisoning from the bug spray.

2. Immediate treatment priorities include:
    *   Scene safety
    *   Consider barrier devices for your personal protection
    *   Initial assessment to include airway, breathing, circulation, and assessment of LOC
    *   Identify poison substance
    *   Contact medical control as soon as possible
    *   Assess the husband for signs/symptoms of exposure to the poison

3. It is vital to involve the medical control physician in the management decisions used in caring for this patient. This is necessary so that the physician can contact the Poison Control Center for treatment guidelines. The physician can also direct the primary and secondary care of the patient at the scene with you, the EMT, functioning as his or her eyes, ears, and hands.

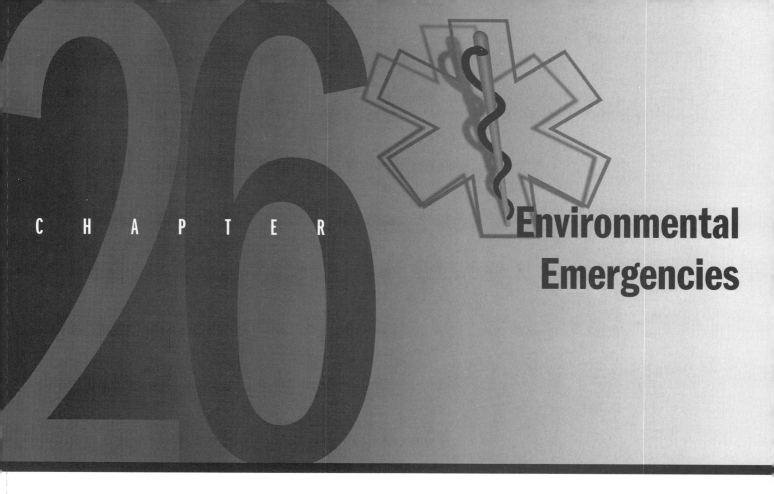

C H A P T E R

Environmental Emergencies

Reading Assignment: Chapter 26, pgs. 418–441

OBJECTIVES

1. Describe the ways the body loses heat.

2. List the signs and symptoms of general and local exposure to cold.

3. List the signs and symptoms of general and local exposure to heat.

4. Detail the steps of emergency care for the patient exposed to cold or heat.

5. Identify the signs and symptoms of water-related emergencies.

6. Describe the complications of near drowning.

7. Describe the emergency medical treatment of bites and stings.

INTRODUCTION

Recognizing signs and symptoms and implementing proper treatment for exposure patients are essential goals in the care of environmental emergencies. This chapter describes how the body regulates and maintains its internal or core temperature, and the various ways heat is lost by the body through such processes as convection, conduction, evaporation, and radiation. The information in the chapter also discusses the external and internal effect(s) on patients from prolonged exposure to either a hot or cold environment.

The chapter describes signs and symptoms of environmental emergencies, from thermal injuries, cold injuries, drowning, and near drowning to and bites and stings. In addition, the chapter addresses prehospital management of patients affected by environmental emergencies.

REVIEW QUESTIONS

Please circle one correct answer for each question.

1. The body continuously attempts to maintain its internal temperature. Major compensatory mechanisms of the body to release heat include: (C 4-7.1)

   a. peripheral vasodilation
   b. sweating
   c. increased respiratory rate
   d. all of the above

2. The conversion of food to energy is called: (C 4-7.1)

   a. metabolism
   b. homeostasis
   c. circulation
   d. glycolysis

3. A regular body temperature (oral) for healthy people is: (C 4-7.9)

   a. 39°C
   b. 98.6°F
   c. 96.8°F
   d. 32°C

4. Most of the time, the body is cooler than the surrounding air. (C 4-7.9)

   a. true
   b. false

5. When the amount of heat gain is greater than the amount of heat given off, higher than normal core temperature exists. This condition is called: (C 4-7.1)

   a. hypothermia
   b. hyperthermia
   c. hypovolemia
   d. hypernatremia

6. The body is warmed by the evaporation of sweat. (C 4-7.1)

   a. true
   b. false

7. _____ is the direct heat exchange that occurs when two or more different temperature surfaces come into direct contact. (C 4-7.1)

   a. Convection
   b. Evaporation
   c. Radiation
   d. Conduction

8. After exposure to cold, the blood vessels closer to the skin surface will _____. This process allows less heat to escape from the body through the skin surface, causing the body's core to stay warmer. (C 4-7.1)

    a. constrict
    b. narrow
    c. dilate
    d. a and b

9. Environmental factors that can affect how well the body will maintain its core temperature include: (C 4-7.1)

    a. ambient temperature
    b. wind
    c. humidity and heat index
    d. all of the above

10. High humidity levels hinder the evaporation of sweat from the skin surface. (C 4-7.4)

    a. true
    b. false

11. Exposure to a cold environment can create a condition known as _____: (C 4-7.2)

    a. hypothermia
    b. hyperthermia
    c. hypovolemia
    d. hypernatremia

12. Factors that can predispose a patient to hypothermia include all of the following **except**: (C 4-7.2)

    a. the patient's age
    b. medical conditions
    c. the use of alcohol or drugs
    d. increased heart rate

13. Head and/or spinal cord injury can affect the central nervous system and alter the body's ability to control internal temperature. (C 4-7.4)

    a. true
    b. false

14. Medical conditions may contribute to the body's ability to regulate its internal temperature. These disorders include all the following **except**: (C 4-7.2)

    a. diabetes
    b. hypoglycemia
    c. hypertension
    d. central nervous system (CNS) disorders

15. Skin condition may help show the extent and/or phase of the cold exposure. Changes in skin color usually progress in the following order: (C 4-7.2)

    a. blue, pale, red
    b. red, pale, blue
    c. pale, blue, red
    d. red, blue, pale

16. Signs or symptoms to look for in possible environmental emergencies include all of the following **except**: (C 4-7.6)

    a. changes in the level of consciousness or mental status
    b. poor coordination, memory disturbances, reduced sense of touch or sensation
    c. mood changes, an increase in normal level of communication abilities and good judgment
    d. dizziness and speech difficulties

17. Treatment of the localized cold-exposed patient includes all of the following **except**: (C 4-7.3)

    a. remove the patient from the environment as safely and as rapidly as possible
    b. protect the cold injured extremity or tissue from further injury
    c. do not remove wet or restricting clothing
    d. administer oxygen

18. Different categories of localized cold exposure include: (C 4-7.2)

    a. frostnip
    b. frostbite
    c. deep frostbite
    d. all of the above

19. The most serious category of localized cold exposure is: (C 4-7.2)

    a. frostnip
    b. frostbite
    c. deep frostbite
    d. all of the above

20. A slow heart rate is very common in the hypothermic patient. (C 4-7.2)

    a. true
    b. false

21. The cold-exposed patient must be handled gently. Rough handling (even CPR) may cause the patient to go into: (C 4-7.3)

    a. a cardiac dysrhythmia
    b. ventricular fibrillation
    c. hyperthermia
    d. a and b

22. All of the following are true statements regarding heat stroke **except**: (C 4-7.4)

    a. it is a true life-threatening emergency
    b. results from the failure of the body's heat-regulating mechanisms
    c. the body is able to cool itself and the core temperature is hypothermic
    d. most cases of heat stroke occur on hot, humid days

23. The patient exposed to heat should be managed by: (C 4-7.5, 10)

    a. removal from the hot environment as safely as possible
    b. placing in a cooler environment, such as the patient compartment of the air-conditioned ambulance
    c. loosening or removing clothing and fanning the patient
    d. all of the above

24. General characteristics of superficial or first degree burns include: (C 5-2.12, 13)

    a. reddened skin
    b. no blisters (open and/or closed) present
    c. patient will complain of localized pain
    d. all of the above

25. General characteristics of partial thickness burns or second degree burns include: (C 5-2.14, 15)

    a. reddening of the skin
    b. blister(s) (open and/or closed) present
    c. patient will complain of localized pain
    d. all of the above

26. In dealing with burns, recognize that charring of the skin and tissue damage through the skin to underlying tissues are general characteristics of: (C 5-2.16, 17)

    a. full-thickness burns or third degree burns
    b. superficial or first degree burns
    c. partial-thickness or second degree burns
    d. superficial and partial-thickness burns

27. The percentage of body surface area (BSA) involved in burns is generally measured using the rule of nines. For a rough estimation of the BSA involved in a burn, the palmar area of the patient will cover approximately _% of the patient's BSA. (C 5-2.11)

    a. 1
    b. 2
    c. 3
    d. 4

28. Local protocols generally dictate which burns are considered critical burns. A burn may be classified as critical if it involves which of the following areas of the patient's body: (C 5-2.11)

    a. hands
    b. feet
    c. genitals
    d. all of the above

29. Cover partial and full thickness burns with moist sterile dressings unless greater than 9% of the patient's body is burned. (P 5-2.36, 37, 38)

    a. true
    b. false

30. _____ is defined as death by asphyxia after submersion. (C 4-7.6)

    a. Drowning
    b. Near drowning
    c. Suffocation
    d. Submersion

31. If the patient is known to have had a diving accident, or if it is uncertain, always suspect an injury and protect the spine. (C 4-7.6)

    a. true
    b. false

32. The overall treatment of any near drowning patient includes all of the following **except**: (C 4-7.11)

   a. allow the patient to go home if he or she is stable
   b. protect and maintain the airway
   c. ventilate the patient if necessary
   d. retain body heat and transport the patient

33. Patients who have been submerged and who are now alert and responsive should still be evaluated by a doctor due to the tremendous potential for complications. (C 4-7.7, 11)

   a. true
   b. false

34. The EMT should examine all injection sites for the presence of a stinger. If a stinger is still visible at the injection site, he or she should: (C 4-7.8)

   a. remove it by scraping along the skin with the edge of a stiff card
   b. use tweezers or forceps to remove the stinger
   c. never attempt to remove the stinger in the field
   d. cover the stinger with a sterile dressing

35. Management of the patient who has been the victim of an animal bite includes: (C 4-7.8)

   a. gently wash the area
   b. remove jewelry from the injured extremity before swelling begins
   c. place the bite site below the patient's heart level
   d. all of the above

Scenario

Read each scenario. Write the answers to the corresponding questions in the space provided.

SCENARIO #1:

You and your partner receive a call to a local service station. Upon arrival, you are led by the station attendant to a 35-year-old male, lying prone on the ground beside a late model car. The attendant tells you that the patient was knocked to the ground when he opened the radiator cap. Steam is billowing from the raised hood on the car. The patient is conscious, alert, and complaining of pain in his right arm, right side, and face.

Upon initial assessment, you find large patches of reddened skin, with evidence of blisters. You note that the patient is exhibiting respiratory distress and has obvious swelling about the lips and face.

1. What is your first priority at this scene?

_____

_____

_____

_____

continued

2. List the steps for management of this patient.

_____

_____

_____

_____

3. What are the exposure possibilities in this scenario?

_____

_____

_____

_____

CHAPTER 26 ANSWERS TO REVIEW QUESTIONS

1. d	8. d	15. b	22. c	29. a
2. a	9. d	16. c	23. d	30. a
3. b	10. a	17. c	24. d	31. a
4. b	11. a	18. d	25. d	32. a
5. b	12. d	19. c	26. a	33. a
6. b	13. a	20. a	27. a	34. a
7. d	14. c	21. d	28. d	35. d

SCENARIO SOLUTIONS

Scenario #1

1. Your first priority is scene safety and personal safety.

2. Steps for managing this patient include:
   - C-spine stabilization
   - Assessment of the airway
   - Exposure of the patient's back for a "quick-look" assessment
   - Log roll the patient to the backboard
   - Re-evaluate LOC
   - Assess breathing rate and quality
   - Apply high-flow oxygen
   - Assess circulation
   - Load the patient into the ambulance and rapidly transport
   - Place the patient on humidified oxygen
   - Apply dry, sterile dressings to burn areas
   - Perform a detailed physical exam
   - Notify receiving hospital of your estimated time of arrival
   - Continually reassess airway for complications due to steam/smoke inhalation

3. The possible exposures are heat and exposure to chemicals from the radiator.

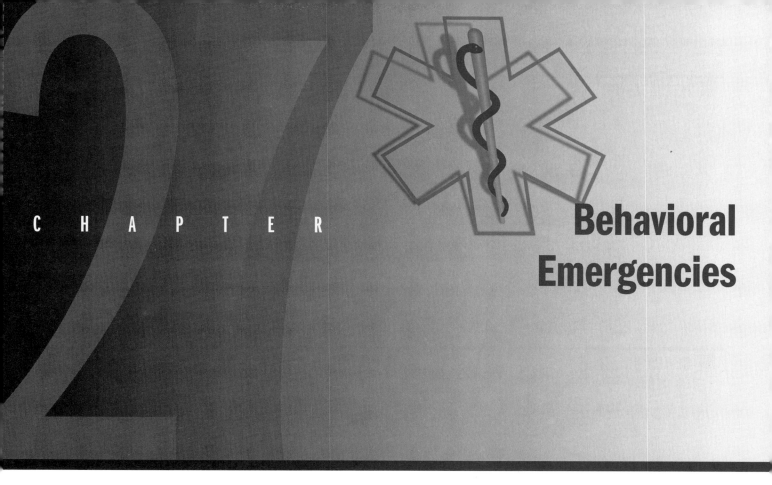

Behavioral Emergencies

C H A P T E R 27

Reading Assignment: Chapter 27, pgs. 442–458

OBJECTIVES

1. State the questions to be considered in assessing a behavioral emergency.

2. List three major causes of behavioral emergencies.

3. Define behavioral emergency.

4. List risk factors for potential suicide.

5. List warning signs of potential suicide.

6. State the medicolegal considerations involved with behavioral and mentally ill patients including those of consent and restraint.

7. Describe assessment of a potentially violent patient, including considerations of past history, posture, vocal activity, and physical activity.

8. Describe management and emergency medical care of a patient undergoing a behavioral emergency.

INTRODUCTION

Patients experiencing behavioral emergencies pose a special situation for prehospital providers. Increasing numbers of individuals, their families, and healthcare agencies call upon the EMS systems when emergency situations present as either a psychologic, inner-perceived crisis or as a disruption of behavior that elicits attention, concern, or upheaval in the immediate environment.

Situations that require immediate recognition and emergency medical intervention include overdoses and self-destructive and homicidal behavior. In view of the often serious outcomes of some behavioral emergencies, it is critical that EMTs dealing with these problems have effective ways of reacting to them. Because EMTs are often the first to arrive at scenes involving persons in a behavioral crisis, this chapter deals with the management of behavioral crises.

REVIEW QUESTIONS

Please circle one correct answer for each question.

1. A behavioral emergency is a reaction to an event that interferes with the daily activities of living. (C 4-8.1)

   a. true
   b. false

2. If the EMT encounters a patient who is experiencing a behavioral emergency and threatening violence, the EMT should: (C 4-8.6)

   a. restrain the patient
   b. leave the immediate area and call the police
   c. call another EMS unit
   d. not interfere

3. You and your crew arrive at a scene where a patient, Mr. Jones, is threatening to kill himself. After you talk with Mr. Jones, he states that he was only joking and will be fine now. You realize that you should: (P 4-8.10)

   a. accept that the patient has dealt with the emergency
   b. wait until his priest arrives, then leave the scene
   c. assume control of the scene and restrain the patient
   d. transport the patient to the hospital for evaluation

4. Authorization to restrain a patient is often provided by: (P 4-8.11)

   a. medical direction
   b. lead medic
   c. any available EMT
   d. clergy

5. Various behaviors may be the result of: (C 4-8.2)

   a. sudden illness or trauma
   b. drug or alcohol intoxication
   c. acute organic brain syndrome
   d. all of the above

6. _____ causes are those behaviors related to mental or psychic factors. (C 4-8.3)
   a. Physiologic
   b. Photogenic
   c. Psychogenic
   d. Philosophic

7. The process of learning to adapt to a variety of situations involving our activities of daily living is called: (C 4-8.2)
   a. alignment
   b. alteration
   c. acclimation
   d. adjustment

8. A mental disorder is: (C 4-8.3)
   a. an illness with psychologic or behavioral manifestations
   b. an impairment in functioning due to social, psychologic, genetic, physical/chemical or biologic disturbance
   c. not limited to relations between the person and society
   d. all of the above

9. All abnormal or disturbing behavior is indicative of mental illness. (C 4-8.2)
   a. true
   b. false

10. When caring for a patient undergoing a behavioral emergency who will not respond to questions, the EMT should observe the patient's emotional state via assessment of: (P 4-8.10)
    a. facial expressions, posture, gestures
    b. pulse and respiratory rates
    c. tears, sweating, or blushing
    d. all of the above

11. In assessing a patient involved in a behavioral emergency, the same initial principles apply as for any other patient. (P 4-8.10)
    a. true
    b. false

12. Assessment of a behavioral emergency includes consideration of the patient's: (P 4-8.10)
    a. orientation and memory
    b. patient responses
    c. level of distraction
    d. all of the above

13. The basic information needed to assess behavioral emergencies requires that the EMT determine the exact causes of the current crisis. (C 4-8.6)
    a. true
    b. false

14. Major causative factors of behavioral emergencies include all of the following **except**: (C 4-8.3)

    a. inadequate cerebral oxygen
    b. drugs
    c. psychogenic circumstances
    d. ability to deal with activities of daily living

15. Patients who are anxious, reluctant, suspicious, and show unnatural fears of what most people would consider normal activities (e.g., walking outside) may be categorized as: (C 4-8.6)

    a. chronically depressed
    b. phobic
    c. always suicidal
    d. probably homicidal

16. The most significant factor contributing to suicide that transcends any other marker is: (C 4-8.4)

    a. depression
    b. phobia
    c. paranoia
    d. anxiety

17. Suicide threats indicate that a person is in a crisis that he or she cannot handle and requires thorough, immediate care. (C 4-8.4)

    a. true
    b. false

18. Risk factors of suicide have been identified as all of the following **except**: (C 4-8.4)

    a. depression, any age
    b. male sex, age over 55
    c. intact, strong emotional bonds
    d. recent loss of spouse, significant other or family member

19. If, during the initial assessment of a patient, you think that suicide is a possibility, you should: (C 4-8.8)

    a. not hesitate to ask the patient questions that may lead to a preliminary assessment
    b. discount the feelings, realizing that the patient is just depressed
    c. ignore vague if offered in a joking context
    d. not bring the subject up because you might be giving the patient ideas

20. Critical warning signs that the patient has a specific suicide plan include: (C 4-8.4)

    a. recently preparation of a will
    b. advising friends what to do with significant possessions
    c. arranging for funeral services
    d. all of the above

21. The EMT should remember that the suicidal patient may be homicidal as well. Management of this patient would include: (A 4-8.9)

a. do nothing either to frighten the patient or to arouse suspicion
b. do not risk your life or the lives of members of your emergency unit
c. police intervention is absolutely required
d. all of the above

22. A standard of care must be carefully adhered to since the patient experiencing a behavioral emergency does not have the ability to make rational decisions about his or her emergency medical care. (C 4-8.5)

a. true
b. false

23. Most states have statutory provisions regarding the emergency care of the mentally ill and drug-dependent persons. These statutory provisions provide certain personnel with the authority to place such a person in protective custody so that emergency care can be rendered. These personnel are: (C 4-8.5)

a. mental health workers
b. human resources agents
c. law enforcement officers
d. emergency medical officers

24. In emergency situations, the implied consent rule applies to the mentally ill patient. This rule generally holds that . . . "If an emergency exists and the patient is unable to give consent, the EMT is able to provide care because implied consent exists." (C 4-8.5)

a. true
b. false

25. When dealing with psychiatric emergencies, it is always clear that a life-threatening emergency exists. (C 4-8.5)

a. true
b. false

26. Cases involving psychiatric crisis should ordinarily involve police intervention. Police involvement provides the: (C 4-8.5)

a. appropriate backup often needed in managing such crisis
b. necessary legal authority to restrain
c. power needed for the EMT to order restraints
d. a and b

27. In the case of potential violence, care must be exercised not only for the patient, but for others in the immediate vicinity. (C 4-8.7)

a. true
b. false

28. When assessing the violent patient, one of the most obvious factors to look for is the _____ activity. (C 4-8.7)

    a. postural
    b. vocal
    c. motor
    d. expressed

29. Factors to take into consideration when evaluating the potential for violence include: (C 4-8.7)

    a. poor impulse control
    b. instability of family structure
    c. inability to keep a steady job
    d. all of the above

30. Emergency medical management of patients experiencing psychiatric emergencies involves: (C 4-8.7)

    a. being prepared to spend time to listen to the patient, and prepare for packaging and transportation
    b. having a definite plan of action and stating your intentions and expectations of the patient
    c. speaking in a low, calm voice is often a quieting influence
    d. all of the above

Scenarios

Read each scenario. Write the answers to the corresponding questions in the space provided.

SCENARIO #1:

This has been one of those days. Before completing the PCR from your tenth call, you and your crew receive a call from dispatch regarding a woman who is quite agitated. She is crying and tells you that her boyfriend has threatened to murder her children and then slay himself. She describes him as being "much drunker than usual" and accounts to you that he is pointing his gun at her and her children. He reportedly stated that his boss was driving him crazy and that he just couldn't take it anymore. The woman then begins to scream and drops the telephone. You can make no further contact with her.

Realizing that things **can** always get worse in the EMS business, you and your partner jump into your unit and head for the address, all the while discussing your plan of action.

1. What is the most likely dilemma with this patient?

2. What are the types of behavioral emergencies described in this scenario?

continued

3. How should the EMT handle this situation initially?

    _____

    _____

    _____

    _____

SCENARIO #2:

It is a quiet Sunday morning. You and your EMT crew are conducting your daily check of your ambulance. Suddenly the emergency tone sounds and you have the distinct impression that your day is about to become interesting! The dispatcher sends you across town to a call from a distressed mother.

En route you learn that a woman has called for help with her 16-year-old daughter. She related that she awoke to find her daughter sitting in the bathtub, fully dressed, rocking back and forth and staring into the distance. She reports that her daughter has not been sleeping well for several weeks now and that she has been depressed.

Upon arrival at the house, you are led to the bathroom where the patient is found just as the mother described. The mother goes on to tell you that she found a note in her daughter's room that detailed her wishes for her funeral arrangements. Sarah has recently stated that she was abandoning her plans for college. When asked to speak to you, the teenager did not reply. She merely continued to gaze away and remains expressionless.

1. What do you think the problem is here?

    _____

    _____

    _____

    _____

2. What are the indications that this patient is experiencing a behavioral emergency?

    _____

    _____

    _____

    _____

3. How should you deal with this patient?

    _____

    _____

    _____

    _____

CHAPTER 27 ANSWERS TO REVIEW QUESTIONS

1. a	6. c	11. a	17. a	24. a
2. b	5. d	10. d	16. a	23. c
3. d	4. a	9. b	15. b	22. a
4. a	10. d	8. d	14. d	21. d
5. d	11. a	7. d	13. b	20. d
6. c	12. d		18. c	19. a

SCENARIOS SOLUTIONS

Scenario #1:

1. This patient is experiencing a major life interruption and is obviously having an acute emotional and mental breakdown. His behavior is not within the normal range of response. Assessment of his behavior suggests some form of mental disorder.
2. This individual is exhibiting both suicidal and homicidal behavior.
3. This patient poses a danger to all persons coming into contact with him, including EMTs. Remember scene safety and personal safety are the primary concerns. The EMTs should not enter this scene; rather they should immediately call for law enforcement intervention.

Scenario #2:

1. This patient is depressed and is at risk for suicide.
2. The withdrawal from reality, as exhibited by this patient, often precedes suicide attempts. The detailed writing of funeral arrangements indicates preparation to die. Depression is a major factor in suicide ideology.
3. You should continue to attempt to talk with this patient in a calm manner and advocate that the patient go to the hospital. If the patient refuses, law enforcement assistance should be requested.

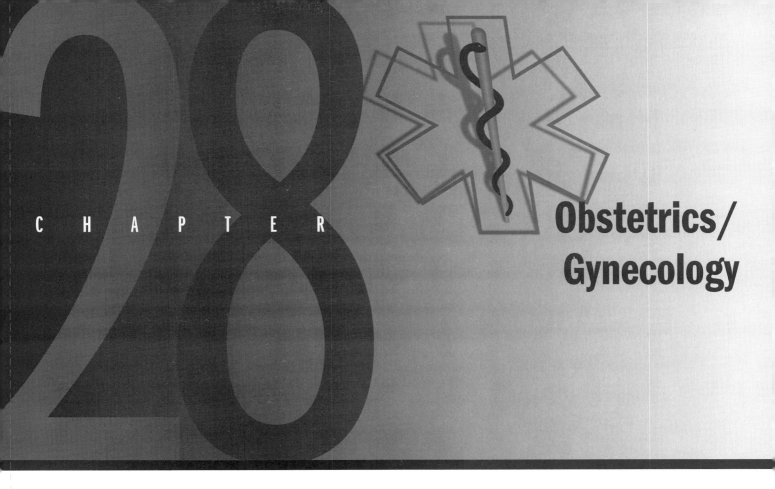

Reading Assignment: Chapter 28, pgs. 459–487

OBJECTIVES

1. Describe the function of the following structures: uterus, vagina, fetus, placenta, umbilical cord, amniotic sac, amniotic fluid, and the perineum.

2. Demonstrate the use of BSI precautions in dealing with the obstetric or gynecologic patient.

3. Identify and describe the use of the equipment in an obstetric kit.

4. Identify and describe appropriate care for patients with predelivery and gynecological emergencies.

5. Identify indications for imminent delivery and state the steps necessary in the predelivery preparation of the mother.

6. Identify and describe the care needed for a normal vaginal delivery, a multiple birth delivery, a breech delivery, a prolapsed cord delivery, a limb delivery, a meconium delivery, and a premature delivery.

7. Describe the necessary steps for the care of the baby as the head appears.

8. Describe the technique and appropriate time to cut the umbilical cord and the steps necessary for the delivery and transport of the placenta.

9. List the steps in the emergency medical care of the mother after delivery.

10. Summarize neonatal resuscitation procedures.

INTRODUCTION

Facilitating the entrance of a new life into the world can be a rewarding, somewhat intimidating experience for the new EMT. In this chapter, the EMT realizes the importance of assessment of the pregnant and non-pregnant woman, and prehospital delivery concerns. This chapter also includes a discussion of appropriate prehospital treatment.

The definition of obstetrics is the branch of medicine that deals with the management of women during pregnancy, childbirth, and 42 days after the expulsion of all contents of pregnancy. Gynecology is defined as the study of the diseases of the female reproductive organs. This chapter discusses birth and the birthing process, the problems associated with pregnancy, the care of newborns, and the care necessary for the person who may have been sexually assaulted.

REVIEW QUESTIONS

Please circle one correct answer for each question.

1. It is important to realize that in all women of reproductive age (from 9 to 55 years old), pregnancy is a very real possibility. (A 4-9.19)

    (a) true
    b. false

2. A primary function of the ovaries is the release of eggs and hormones. Normally, one ovary releases a mature egg once a month in a process known as: (C 4-9.1)

    a. fertilization
    b. flatulation
    (c) ovulation
    d. menopause

3. You are dispatched to a woman who is 8 months pregnant. Her husband summons the EMS service because his wife has suddenly developed massive vaginal bleeding. You should consider all of the following actions **except**: (C 4-9.5)

    a. administer high-flow oxygen
    (b) walk patient to the ambulance and transport
    c. place her on the stretcher with her legs elevated
    d. transport immediately

4. The process in which the lining of the uterus is shed when the egg is not fertilized is known as: (C 4-9.1)

    a. ovulation
    b. menstruation
    c. ministration
    d. fertilization

5. A sexual assault victim should be discouraged from bathing or changing clothes before being transported to the hospital. (C 4-9.18)

    a. true
    b. false

6. If both ovaries are damaged, removed, or have stopped producing matured eggs, a female will go through a process called: (C 4-9.1)

    a. menopause
    b. ovulation
    c. menstruation
    d. fertilization

7. If a fertilized egg implants in a fallopian tube, it will grow until the fallopian tube ruptures. This condition is known as a tubal (ectopic) pregnancy and can threaten the mother's life. (C 4-9.1)

    a. true
    b. false

8. The _____ houses the unborn baby during fetal development. (C 4-9.1)

    a. vagina
    b. cervix
    c. umbilicus
    d. uterus

9. In the last 3 months of pregnancy, the uterus becomes heavy due to the weight of the fetus. Lying on the back at this stage of pregnancy can restrict the circulation of blood to the placenta because the uterus will be resting on the mother's: (C 4-9.1)

    a. inferior vena cava
    b. superior vena cava
    c. amniotic sac
    d. placenta

10. The _____ is a fibromuscular sheath that encloses the lower end of the uterus. (C 4-9.1)

    a. vagina
    b. anus
    c. urethra
    d. orifice

11. The vagina is also known as the: (C 4-9.1)

    a. amniotic sac
    b. birth canal
    c. perineum
    d. tetial site

12. Between the eighth week of development and delivery, the embryo is known as a(n): (C 4-9.1)

    a. fetus
    b. egg
    c. uterus
    d. placenta

13. The placenta exchanges oxygen and carbon dioxide between fetus and mother, transports nutrients and waste by-products, and serves as a temporary source for hormone production necessary to sustain the pregnancy. (C 4-9.1)

    a. true
    b. false

14. The umbilical cord is a fibrous, whitish tube that connects the baby to the: (C 4-9.1)

    a. placenta
    b. umbilical cord
    c. vessels
    d. umbilical vein

15. Once the embryo is imbedded in the uterus, a protective covering completely surrounds the embryo, known as the: (C 4-9.1)

    a. amniotic sac
    b. mucous plug
    c. umbilical cord
    d. placenta

16. The _____ stage of labor begins with the full dilation of the cervix and ends with the delivery of the baby. (P 4-9.20)

    a. first
    b. second
    c. third
    d. fourth

17. The part of the infant that protrudes initially is called the: (P 4-9.20)

    a. presenting part
    b. shoulder
    c. buttocks
    d. appendage

18. The visualization of the presenting part is commonly referred to as: (P 4-9.20)

    a. third stage
    b. condensing
    c. crowning
    d. contracting

19. Appropriate equipment is essential for an organized delivery. The contents of a delivery kit should include all of the following components **except**: (C 4-9.2)

    a. surgical scissors, hemostats, cord clamps
    b. umbilical tape, bulb syringe, towels
    c. gauze sponges, forceps, Valium, nonsterile gloves
    d. baby blankets, sanitary napkins, plastic bag

20. An embryo or fetus that is expelled from the uterus before week 20, whether by nature or choice, is classified as a(n): (C 4-9.3)

   a. abortion
   b. miscarriage
   c. placenta previa
   d. a and b

21. Bleeding in the last 3 months of pregnancy is an unusual situation. If bleeding does occur, the patient should be: (C 4-9.5)

   a. placed on high-flow oxygen
   b. transported to the hospital as quickly as possible
   c. if exhibiting signs of shock, treat the symptoms of shock
   d. all of the above

22. One type of late vaginal bleeding is known as _____ _____, and is caused by the sudden separation of the placenta from the wall of the uterus. (C 4-9.3)

   a. abruptio placentae
   b. vaginal bleeding
   c. placenta previa
   d. placenta implantation

23. Treatment for patients with abruptio placentae and placenta previa consists of: (P 4-9.27)

   a. maintaining an open airway
   b. administering high-flow oxygen via nonrebreather mask
   c. treating the symptoms of shock by placing the patient in a supine position and elevating the legs
   d. all of the above

24. During delivery, BSI must be maintained. Protective eyewear is essential. (C 4-9.7)

   a. true
   b. false

25. Sometimes prehospital delivery is imminent, and the EMT must be prepared to deliver the baby. All of the following are signs that the EMT must prepare for delivery **except**: (C 4-9.4)

   a. the beginning of one contraction to the beginning of the next contraction is between 6 and 9 minutes in length
   b. contractions that are regular and lasting from 45 to 60 seconds
   c. the woman in later pregnancy who wants to go to the bathroom to move her bowels
   d. the mother wants to bear down or push

26. For optimum care it is recommended that each patient (mother and baby) will need at least one EMT. (P 4-9.19)

   a. true
   b. false

27. Steps in the predelivery preparation of the mother include: (C 4-9.6)

   a. have the mother lie on her back, knees drawn up, and spread apart and elevate the patient's buttocks with a blanket

   b. create a sterile field around the vaginal opening using sterile towels or sterile packaged paper drapes

   c. make sure that enough space exists in front of the mother at the end of the stretcher or bed

   d. all of the above

28. With each contraction, the vaginal opening bulges to accommodate the delivery of the head. The EMT should: (C 4-9.8, 9)

   a. place a gloved hand on the presenting part

   b. exert slight pressure to prevent an explosive delivery

   c. once the head has emerged from the vaginal opening, examine the infant's neck for a loop of umbilical cord

   d. all of the above

29. If the looped umbilical cord can be gently slipped over the infant's head, this should be done. If the looped umbilical cord cannot be slipped over the infant's head, the EMT should: (C 4-9.10)

   a. clamp the umbilical cord in three places

   b. place ties between the clamps

   c. clamp the umbilical cord in two places

   d. leave the cord around the infant's neck

30. The placenta is expelled from the vagina after delivery. The average time for the delivery of the placenta is approximately __ minutes after the delivery of the infant. (C 4-9.11)

   a. 10

   b. 20

   c. 15

   d. 30

31. Continuing assessment of the mother postdelivery is as important as continuing assessment of the newborn. If the mother is in shock, regardless of the amount of blood lost, the mother should be treated for shock with: (C 4-9)

   a. supplemental oxygen

   b. proper positioning

   c. rapid transport to the hospital

   d. all of the above

32. A scoring system has been instituted to evaluate the condition of the infant after 1 minute and 5 minutes of life. This scoring system is called the: (C 4-9.13)

   a. AVPU score

   b. AUPV score

   c. Apgar score

   d. AMGAR score

33. Newborns who need resuscitation have problems with either airway, breathing, or circulation. If one of these situations occurs the EMT should: (C 4-9.13)

   a. warm and dry the infant
   b. position and suction the infant
   c. stimulate the infant
   d. all of the above

34. Meconium in the amniotic fluid indicates fetal distress. It is important to clear the infant's airway of meconium with suction when it is born, otherwise a severe _____ problem may occur. (C 4-9.16)

   a. cardiovascular
   b. circulatory
   c. respiratory
   d. hepatic

35. In a breech birth, the presenting part is the: (C 4-9.14)

   a. buttocks of the fetus
   b. foot or leg of the fetus
   c. head of the fetus
   d. a or b

36. Situations in which the EMT inserts a gloved hand into the vagina are: (C 4-9.14)

   a. prolapsed cord
   b. lower body or leg breech delivery
   c. shoulder or hand delivery
   d. all of the above

37. A patient delivering twins should have _ EMTs at the scene. (C 4-9.15)

   a. 2
   b. 4
   c. 3
   d. 1

38. Multiple births are at risk for premature deliveries. (C 4-9.15)

   a. true
   b. false

39. Premature babies are always at risk for: (C 4-9.17)

   a. rapid heart rate
   b. rapid body heat loss
   c. slow body heat loss
   d. rapid dehydration

40. A pregnant trauma victim should be transported even though the injury appears to be minor. Adequate resuscitation of the mother is the key to survival of the mother and fetus. (C 4-9.26)

   a. true
   b. false

Scenarios

Read each scenario. Write the answers to the corresponding questions in the space provided.

SCENARIO #1:

Your day has been a real test of your dedication to EMS! Its definitely been one of those "Murphy's Law" days and you are not at all sad that your shift ends in only 15 minutes . . . you KNOW that tomorrow will be a better day!

Suddenly, the emergency phone rings and you realize that indeed your day is not over yet. Dispatch directs you to a residence where you and your partner find a pregnant female who states that she is 9 months pregnant. Upon initial assessment, you quickly learn that she is a multipara, as this is her seventh pregnancy. Now you know for sure that tomorrow has to be a better day!

As you examine the patient, you find that her contractions are 1-2 minutes apart and she is bearing down, all the while begging to be allowed to go to the bathroom. You and your partner immediately set up for delivery at home. Moments later, the baby is crowning. You note that the umbilical cord is wrapped around the baby's neck.

1. How would you handle this situation?

   _____

   _____

   _____

   _____

2. List the equipment and state the purpose of each piece of equipment needed to handle this emergency home delivery.

   _____

   _____

   _____

   _____

continued

SCENARIO #2:

You and your EMT crew have had a busy day and, as you joked about earlier, there is a beautiful moon out tonight. Sure enough, just as you sit down to dinner, you receive a call to a rural address, approximately 15 miles from the station. Dispatch notifies you that the call came in from a frantic man who stated that his wife is "very pregnant" and is suddenly ill.

En route to the scene, you and your partner discuss your plan of action and decide never to joke about a full moon again! Upon arrival you find a 35 year old female who is visibly pregnant and says that her due date is next week. The patient denies pain, but states that she is experiencing bright red bleeding that started about 15 minutes ago. She is anxious and tells you that this is her first pregnancy.

Upon initial assessment and physical examination, you find that your patient is pale and her skin is moist and cool to touch. Assessment of vital signs reveals B/P = 90/60, heart rate = 134, and respirations = 30. Heart sounds are well heard and breath sounds are clear. Fetal heart sounds are audible.

1.   What are your conclusions based on the patient's vital signs?

_____

_____

_____

_____

2.   List the steps of management of this patient.

_____

_____

_____

_____

3.   What is the medical term(s) for this patient's condition?

_____

_____

_____

_____

4.   Differentiate between placenta previa and abruptio placenta.

_____

_____

_____

_____

CHAPTER 28 ANSWERS TO REVIEW QUESTIONS

1.	a	9.	a	17.	a	25.	a	33.	d
2.	c	10.	a	18.	c	26.	a	34.	c
3.	b	11.	b	19.	c	27.	d	35.	d
4.	b	12.	a	20.	d	28.	d	36.	d
5.	a	13.	a	21.	d	29.	a	37.	c
6.	a	14.	a	22.	a	30.	b	38.	a
7.	a	15.	a	23.	d	31.	d	39.	b
8.	d	16.	b	24.	a	32.	c	40.	a

SCENARIOS SOLUTIONS

Scenario #1:

1. You should gently try to unwrap the cord from the baby's neck. This maneuver will be successful in most cases. If your manual manipulation of the cord doesn't work, you must immediately clamp the cord and cut it.

2. Prepackaged equipment is essential for a successful and organized delivery. The contents of a delivery kit should include the following components:

- Surgical Scissors: used for cutting the cord.
- Hemostats or cord clamp: used for clamping the cord.
- Umbilical tape or sterilized cord: used for tying off the placenta side of the umbilical cord.
- Bulb syringe: used for suctioning the mouth and nose of the infant.
- Towels: used for drying and stimulating the infant.
- Gauze sponges, 2×10 : used to clear secretions from the infant's mouth and to pat the ends of the cut umbilical cord.
- Sterile gloves: used for BSI for the EMT.
- Baby Blanket (1): used to keep the baby warm.
- Sanitary Napkins: used to absorb the drainage of blood from the vagina.
- Plastic Bag: used as a receptacle for transporting the placenta.

The kit should be packaged in a moisture-resistant receptacle with a date of expiration to prevent deterioration of the contents.

Scenario #2:

1. You realize that the patient's airway is patent as she is breathing without distress. Her respirations are a bit rapid and you realize that this could be caused by anxiety and is probably the body's compensatory mechanism for coping with blood loss. Her circulation is being maintained, but is compromised because the patient's heart rate is rapid and her B/P is lower than it should be at this stage of pregnancy. The fact that, at this point, she is able to answer all questions appropriately indicates adequate perfusion to the brain. You should have a high index of suspicion of impending shock, based on the current vital signs. You realize that her vital signs must be monitored carefully during transport.

2. You should:

    a. Immediately institute body substance isolation.

    b. Realize that it is inappropriate to perform a vaginal examination on a woman with third trimester bleeding.

    c. Proceed to do a *visual* examination of the patient's perineal area, making sure that your partner is in the room. Upon examination of the patient's perineum, you note a moderate amount of bright red blood oozing from the vaginal opening.

    d. Without delay, instruct your partner to place the mother on high-flow oxygen using a nonrebreather mask with reservoir.

    e. Notify dispatch to summon an ALS unit, if available, to the scene, as the patient needs volume replacement via intravenous infusions.

    f. Tilt the patient to her left side.

    g. Transport the patient to the hospital as rapidly and safely as possible.

    h. Notify the hospital of your ETA so that they can be prepared for your arrival and can summon the patient's obstetrician to the hospital to attend the patient.

3. This patient is probably presenting with placenta previa. It is difficult to distinguish clinically between placenta previa and abruptio placenta. There are, however, certain features of this patient's case that suggest the former.

4. In abruptio placenta, there is more likely to be pain related bleeding. Bright red blood is more characteristic of placenta previa. The passage of dark blood is more common with abruptio placenta. You realize that both conditions may be rapidly fatal. It is not important in the field to distinguish between the two conditions. All cases of third-trimester bleeding should be considered a medical emergency; the patient should be treated accordingly.

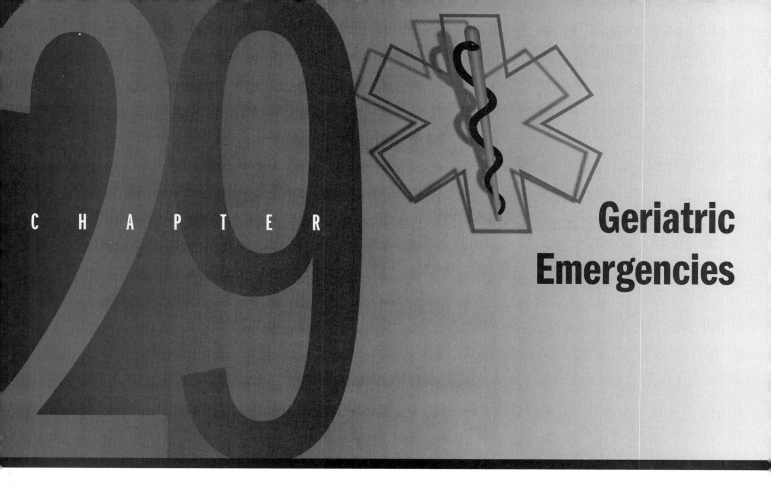

CHAPTER 29

Geriatric Emergencies

Reading Assignment: Chapter 29, pgs. 488–506

OBJECTIVES

1. Define the term "elderly."
2. State the leading causes of death of the elderly.
3. Describe the process of gathering patient information for the elderly person.
4. List the steps in assessing an elderly patient.
5. Describe communication basics used with an elderly patient.
6. Describe trauma assessment in the elderly.
7. Describe acute illness assessment in the elderly.
8. State the nature of the problem of elder abuse.
9. List the categories and characteristics of elder abuse.

INTRODUCTION

Elderly patients currently represent approximately 11% of the population of the United States. This represents approximately 26 million persons. By the year 2030, it is estimated that the elderly will represent approximately 18% of the United States population. The term elderly typically refers to persons 65 years of age and older.

Since the elderly represent the fastest growing age group in the nation, this chapter explains the general techniques of assessment, communication, and management when dealing with elderly patients. The elderly present EMTs with notable emergency medical care management challenges.

REVIEW QUESTIONS

Please circle one correct answer for each question.

1. In the elderly patient category, the leading cause of death is: (Chp. Obj. #2)

   a. cancer
   b. cardiovascular disease
   c. diabetes
   d. trauma

2. Changes caused by the aging process in physical structure, body composition, and organ function often affect emergency medical care. (Chp. Obj. #4)

   a. true
   b. false

3. The elderly are considered at high risk for many mental health problems. (Chp. Obj. #7)

   a. true
   b. false

4. The term elderly is not necessarily age specific. Patients who are ___ years of age and older are by definition, considered to be elderly. (Chp. Obj. #1)

   a. 50
   b. 45
   c. 65
   d. 70

5. Risk factors affecting the death rate in the elderly include: (Chp. Obj. #3)

   a. being over 75 years of age
   b. living alone and being immobile
   c. recent death of a significant other
   d. all of the above

6. Aging is a natural biological process. Another term for aging is: (Chp. Obj. #1)

   a. pediatric
   b. senescence
   c. juvenile
   d. homeostatic

7. Geriatric patients are a group characterized by all of the following **except:** (Chp. Obj. #1)

   a. frailty, slower mental processes
   b. impairment of psychologic functions, diminished energy
   c. enhancement of psychologic functions, increased energy
   d. advent of degenerative diseases, decline in sensory acuity

8. The well-known superficial signs and symptoms of older age include: (Chp. Obj. #4)

   a. skin wrinkling, changes in hair color and quantity
   b. osteoarthritis
   c. slowness in reaction time
   d. all of the above

9. Bone loss is more rapid in women and accelerates after menopause. Therefore the incidence of _____ is greater in women. (Chp. Obj. #4)

   a. cardiomyopathy
   b. osteoporosis
   c. Parkinson's
   d. prostatitis

10. Older women have a greater probability of fractures, particularly of the: (Chp. Obj. #4)

   a. femur
   b. thigh
   c. foot
   d. a and b

11. Osteoarthritis, a form of arthritis in which joints degenerate, is characterized by: (Chp. Obj. #7)

   a. stiffness
   b. deformity and pain
   c. swelling of the joints
   d. all of the above

12. The cardiac emergency situations that are most consequential in the care of geriatric patients include all of the following **except:** (Chp. Obj. #7)

   a. acute chest pain
   b. dysrhythmia
   c. epiglottitis
   d. coronary artery disease

13. _____ is the name given to a group of diseases characterized by thickening and loss of elasticity of arterial walls. (Chp. Obj. #7)

   a. Osteoporosis
   b. Arteriosclerosis
   c. Obstruction
   d. Arteritis

14. Another risk associated with narrowing and eventual obstruction of the coronary arteries is: (Chp. Obj. #7)

    a. osteoporosis
    b. pericarditis
    c. heart attack
    d. mesenteric infarction

15. In the elderly patient category, the patients may learn more slowly than the young, but once materials are learned, retention is good. (Chp. Obj. #5)

    a. true
    b. false

16. In the prehospital emergency setting, when the elderly are managed for acute illness or trauma, the EMT must be alert to advanced disease states that may cloud initial patient assessment. These include: (Chp. Obj. #6)

    a. failure of the heart to provide adequate circulation
    b. respiratory insufficiency
    c. auditory and visual loss
    d. all of the above

17. Assessment of the elderly in the prehospital environment often takes longer and may be more difficult to conduct due to communication problems such as: (Chp. Obj. #5)

    a. visual impairment
    b. hearing loss
    c. fatigue
    d. all of the above

18. The elderly value factual information and are discerning in evaluating matters based upon their life experiences. The EMT must be aware of all of the following factors **except:** (Chp. Obj. #4)

    a. the elderly desire more privacy
    b. the elderly make quick decisions
    c. they do not respond to directions calling for quick decisions
    d. the sequences of assessment of the elderly may have to be modified because of the presence of sensory deficits

19. Elderly patients may be reluctant to give information without the assistance of a relative or support person. (Chp. Obj. #4)

    a. true
    b. false

20. In trauma assessment, the following must be considered: (Chp. Obj. #6)

    a. airway
    b. dentures
    c. protection of the cervical spine
    d. all of the above

21. Ordinarily, dentures should be left in place because maintaining a seal around the mouth is more difficult without dentures in place. (Chp. Obj. #6)

    a. true
    b. false

22. Degenerative arthritis of the cervical spine may subject the elderly patient to spinal cord injury while maneuvering the neck, even if there is no injury to the spine. (Chp. Obj. #6)

    a. true
    b. false

23. Reports and complaints of abuse of the elderly are reported to be on the rise. The extent of elder abuse is not known for several reasons. These reasons include: (Chp. Obj. #8)

    a. elder abuse has been a problem largely hidden from society
    b. the varying definitions of abuse/neglect in the elderly
    c. the reticence of elders or others to report the problem
    d. all of the above

24. Abuse is defined as any action on the part of an elderly person's family, associated persons who have daily household contact or upon whom the elderly person is reliant for daily needs, or a professional caretaker who takes advantage of the individual's person, property, or emotional state. (Chp. Obj. #8)

    a. true
    b. false

25. The elderly patients most likely to be abused fall into all of the following profiles **except:** (Chp. Obj. #9)

    a. over 45 years of age and male
    b. frail, with multiple chronic medical conditions
    c. dementia and impaired sleep cycle, sleepwalking, shouting
    d. incontinence of feces, urine, or both and dependent upon others for their daily activities of living

26. It is important to remember that many patients suffering abuse are terrorized into making false statements for fear of retribution. (Chp. Obj. #9)

    a. true
    b. false

27. It can be implied, from the data on child abuse, that one preventative measure in reducing maltreatment of the elderly is its identification by emergency medical providers. (Chp. Obj. #9)

    a. true
    b. false

28. Abuse may be categorized as follows: (Chp. Obj. #9)

    a. physical
    b. psychologic
    c. financial
    d. all of the above

29. Detection of geriatric abuse by astute EMS providers may be the single most important factor in its reduction. (Chp. Obj. #6)

    a. true
    b. false

30. The management of geriatric abuse that involves physical violence is always fraught with many concerns. (Chp. Obj. #9)

    a. true
    b. false

Scenario

Read each scenario. Write the answers to the corresponding questions in the space provided.

SCENARIO #1:

You and your partner are dispatched to an exclusive neighborhood in your city to attend a patient who reportedly "fell down." A friend who had dropped by for a visit reported to the E-911 dispatcher that the woman had been quiet and withdrawn for the past few weeks.

Upon arrival at the home, the friend meets you at the ambulance and reports to you that the woman lives with her son who is a successful stock broker. He and his wife travel extensively, but have not been able to place his mother in a nursing home.

You find a 75-year-old female in the kitchen of her son's home. Blood is noted on her face and right arm. Contusions are noted about the face, head, neck, and arms. Initial assessment reveals that the patient is responsive to voice, but appears confused and disoriented.

Her airway is patent and her breathing rate is 18. Her pulse is 72 and her B/P is 170/85. From the appearance of the kitchen, it is obvious that the patient was attempting to prepare a meal for herself.

1. What is your assessment of this scenario?

    _____

    _____

    _____

    _____

2. What might have caused the patient's fall?

    _____

    _____

    _____

    _____

3. How would you attend to this patient?

    _____

    _____

    _____

    _____

4. Is this patient exhibiting signs or symptoms of elderly abuse?

    _____

    _____

    _____

    _____

CHAPTER 29 ANSWERS TO REVIEW QUESTIONS

1. b	7. c	13. b	19. a	25. a
2. a	8. d	14. c	20. d	26. a
3. b	9. b	15. a	21. a	27. a
4. c	10. d	16. d	22. a	28. d
5. d	11. d	17. d	23. d	29. a
6. b	12. c	18. b	24. a	30. a

SCENARIO SOLUTIONS

Scenario #1

1. This patient has obviously been left alone and has been unsuccessful in managing her daily activities. A high index of suspicion of elderly abuse should be foremost in the minds of the attending EMTs.

2. The patient's fall may have been the result of head injury from being battered. It is also possible that the patient may have experienced a physiologic fracture that could have caused her to fall.

3. Since the patient fell down, you should conduct a thorough trauma assessment, including management of ABC and other problems. The patient should be packaged with complete spinal precautions. It would be appropriate to consider the administration of oxygen. It is imperative that this patient be cared for in a calm and efficient manner. She requires transportation to the hospital for further evaluation.

4. Upon arrival at the hospital you should consider notifying the medical staff of the potential problem of elder abuse in this case.

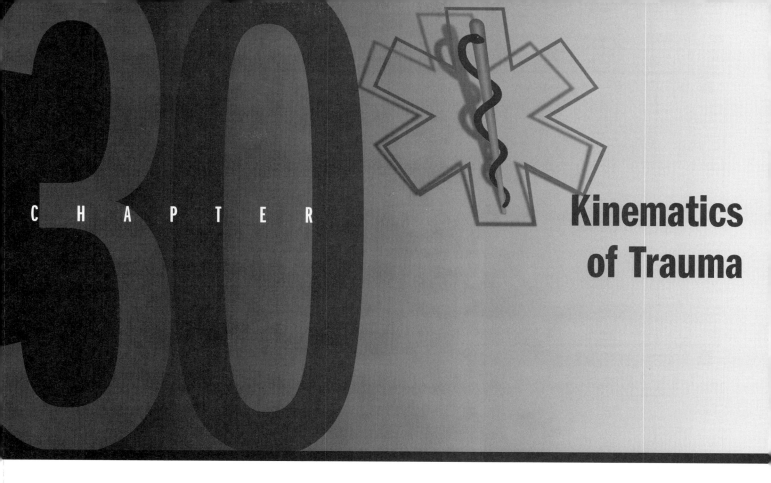

Kinematics of Trauma

Reading Assignment: Chapter 30, pgs. 507–555

OBJECTIVES

1. Define energy and force as they relate to trauma.

2. Define the laws governing motion.

3. Describe the role increased speed plays in causing injuries.

4. Describe each type of auto impact and its effect on unrestrained victims (e.g., "down and under," "up and over," compression, shear).

5. Describe the injuries produced in the head, spine, thorax, and abdomen that result from the various types of automobile collisions.

6. Describe the kinematics of penetrating injuries.

7. Describe the mechanism of energy exchange and the factors that effect speed reduction for a moving body.

8. List the motion and energy considerations of mechanisms other than motor vehicle accidents.

9. Define the role of kinematics as an additional tool for patient assessment.

INTRODUCTION

Treatment of the victims of traumatic injuries depends upon identifying injuries or potential injuries. Good assessment skills are a necessity. This chapter discusses the medical care of the trauma patient as it is divided into three phases: precrash, crash, and postcrash.

The history of a traumatic incident begins in the precrash phase with the events that precede the incident. The second phase in the history of a trauma incident is the crash phase, which begins when one moving object collides with another object. The prehospital provider uses the information gathered about the crash and precrash phases to manage the patient in the postcrash phase.

This chapter provides the information necessary for the EMT to understand the exchange of forces and to translate that information into a prediction of injuries and then into appropriate patient care.

REVIEW QUESTIONS

Please circle one correct answer for each question.

1. _____ first law of motion states that a body at rest will remain at rest and a body in motion will remain in motion unless acted upon by some outside force. (Chp. Obj. #2)

   a. Morton's
   b. Pavlov's
   c. Newton's
   d. Einstein's

2. One principle of physics states that: (Chp. Obj. #2)

   a. energy cannot be created
   b. energy cannot be destroyed
   c. energy can be changed in form
   d. all of the above

3. The motion of a vehicle is a form of energy. When the motion starts or stops the energy must be changed to another form. It may become a form of all of the following types of energy **except:** (Chp. Obj. #2)

   a. mechanical
   b. extrinsic
   c. thermal
   d. chemical

4. All of the following are examples of energy dissipation from an auto accident **except:** (Chp. Obj. #1)

   a. heating of the compressed steel
   b. sound of the impact
   c. internal injury to the vehicle occupant
   d. cooling of the compressed steel

5. The energy of motion can be converted into the heat of friction. This type energy is known as: (Chp. Obj. #1)

   a. thermal energy
   b. chemical energy
   c. mechanical energy
   d. ambient energy

6. Kinetic energy is the energy of _____ and is a function of an object's weight and speed. (Chp. Obj. #2)

   a. sound
   b. light
   c. motion
   d. heat

7. The factor that is considered the most influential when calculating the amount of injury that will be caused by a moving object is the object's: (Chp. Obj. #3)

   a. mass
   b. weight
   c. height
   d. speed

8. Much less damage occurs in a high-speed or high-velocity collision than in a collision at a slower speed. (Chp. Obj. #3)

   a. true
   b. false

9. Although a small child and an adult are different in size and weight, if they are both in a vehicle traveling 65 mph, the most vital determinant of the amount of force that will be applied to them in a crash is their: (Chp. Obj. #3)

   a. common speed, not their weight difference
   b. weight difference, not their common speed
   c. height and weight, not their common speed
   d. height difference, not their common speed

10. An unrestrained driver will be more severely injured than a restrained driver because the restraint system, rather than the body, absorbs a significant portion of the energy of deceleration. (Chp. Obj. #4)

    a. true
    b. false

11. Loss of motion of a moving object can translate into tissue damage to the victim. (Chp. Obj. #4)

    a. true
    b. false

12. Energy exchange is directly related to the density and size of the frontal area at the point of contact between the object and the victim's body. (Chp. Obj. #7)

    a. true
    b. false

13. Shear forces, tearing organs or their supporting structures, come into play with: (Chp. Obj. #4)

    a. deceleration
    b. acceleration
    c. penetrating injuries
    d. a and b

14. In the management of trauma patients, one of the most critical determinates of the outcome is the time from the onset of the injury to the time of: (Chp. Obj. #9)

    a. transport
    b. initial assessment
    c. definitive care
    d. ongoing assessment

15. The difference between blunt and penetrating trauma is whether the skin is actually penetrated. (Chp. Obj. # 6)

    a. true
    b. false

16. In blunt trauma, two forces are involved in the impact. These two forces are: (Chp. Obj. #4)

    a. penetrating injuries
    b. change of speed
    c. compression
    d. b and c

17. Injury can result from any type of impact. Examples of potential injurious impacts include: (Chp. Obj. #8)

    a. a collision on the athletic field
    b. a fall
    c. a pedestrian collision
    d. all of the above

18. When a moving object strikes the human body or when the human body, in motion, strikes a stationary object, the tissue of the human body is knocked out of its normal position. This process is called: (Chp. Obj. #4)

    a. cavitation
    b. penetration
    c. compression
    d. levitation

19. When dealing with the trauma victim, the early identification, adequate understanding, and appropriate treatment of the underlying injury significantly influence whether the patient lives or dies. (Chp. Obj. #9)

    a. true
    b. false

20. Motor vehicle accidents are the most common kinds of blunt trauma, with collisions between pedestrians and motor vehicles a close second. (Chp. Obj. #4)

    a. true
    b. false

21. Part of the job as members of the medical care team is to become active in injury prevention. The EMT should: (Chp. Obj. #9)

    a. strive to be conscientious and informed
    b. educate patients
    c. educate the public regarding prevention
    d. all of the above

22. If a patient has followed a down-and-under path during a frontal collision, the EMT should have a high index of suspicion of all the following injuries **except:** (Chp. Obj. #4)

    a. flail chest
    b. knee dislocations
    c. femur injuries
    d. hip dislocations

23. In the up-and-over motion of a frontal collision, the ____ is usually the lead body portion. (Chp. Obj. #4)

    a. chest
    b. abdomen
    c. head
    d. pelvis

24. A victim involved in a crash as described in Question #23 may have compression injuries to the anterior chest, which may include: (Chp. Obj. #5)

    a. broken ribs
    b. anterior flail chest
    c. pulmonary contusion
    d. all of the above

25. Fractures of the spine are more common with lateral collisions than with rear collisions. (Chp. Obj. #5)

    a. true
    b. false

26. Shear injury to the abdominal organs occurs at their points of attachment to the mesentery. Organs that can shear this way include the: (Chp. Obj. #4)

    a. kidneys
    b. small intestine
    c. the spleen
    d. all of the above

27. Ejection from vehicles accounts for 27% of the 40,000 automobile trauma deaths that occur each year. One out of thirteen ejection victims suffers a: (Chp. Obj. #5)

    a. spinal fracture
    b. hip fracture
    c. pelvic fracture
    d. skull fracture

28. Air bags are extremely effective in the first collision of head-on impacts, but they are not effective in multiple-impact collisions. (Chp. Obj. #9)

    a. true
    b. false

29. The type of motorcyclists' equipment that offers the best protection is: (Chp. Obj. #9)

    a. boots
    b. leather clothing
    c. helmets
    d. all the above

30. In pedestrian collisions, children are initially struck higher on the body than adults. (Chp. Obj. #8)

    a. true
    b. false

Scenario

Read each scenario. Write the answers to the corresponding questions in the space provided.

SCENARIO #1:

You and your partner are called to the scene of a one-vehicle crash. Your patient is a 40-year-old male who reportedly dodged a deer in the road and crashed into a huge oak tree. He is the only occupant in the car. Upon questioning, the patient reluctantly admits that he was not wearing a seat belt.

A quick glance at the car reveals marked damage to the front end. You note a bent steering column and a starburst pattern on the windshield. The patient is conscious and alert. He is restless and anxious.

Initial assessment reveals his heart rate is 128 and his B/P is 86/66. He is respiring adequately at a rate of 28 breaths/min. You note a large bruise on the patient's anterior chest wall.

1. Considering the mechanisms of injury, what injuries should you expect to find?

    _____

    _____

    _____

    _____

2. Of the possible injuries listed above, which one is the most likely contributor to the patient's hypotension?

    _____

    _____

    _____

    _____

3 Does your patient exhibit signs/symptoms of significant hypovolemia? Is so, list at least two signs and/or symptoms.

    _____

    _____

    _____

    _____

CHAPTER 30 ANSWERS TO REVIEW QUESTIONS

1. c	7. d	13. d	19. a	25. a
2. d	8. b	14. c	20. a	26. d
3. b	9. a	15. a	21. d	27. a
4. d	10. a	16. d	22. a	28. b
5. a	11. a	17. d	23. c	29. c
6. c	12. a	18. a	24. d	30. a

SCENARIO SOLUTIONS

Scenario #1

1. The list of possible injuries that you might expect includes:
   - Head: Possible skull fracture(s), cerebral contusion, and increased intracranial pressure.
   - Spine: Possible spinal fracture.
   - Chest: Rib fracture(s), flail chest, cardiac contusion, pneumothorax, and pulmonary contusion.
   - Abdomen: Rending of the liver and/or spleen with possible associated injury to the pancreas.
   - Extremities: Dislocation/fracture of the knee, fracture of the femur or dislocation of the hip.

2. The most likely contributors to the patient's hypovolemia are a ruptured spleen and/or liver.

3. Yes, this patient does exhibit signs/symptoms of hypovolemia. Signs or symptoms of hypovolemia are hypotension, tachycardia, anxiety.

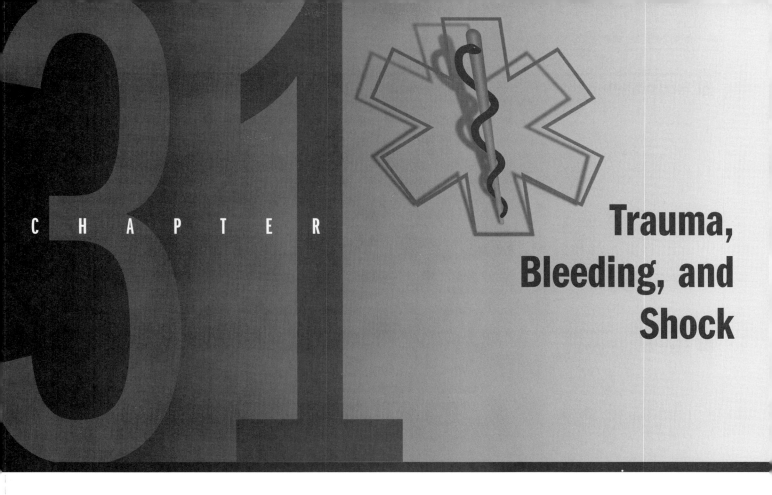

CHAPTER 31

Trauma, Bleeding, and Shock

Reading Assignment: Chapter 31, pgs. 556–576

OBJECTIVES

1. Describe the structure and function of the circulatory system and its most important structures: heart, arteries, veins and capillaries.

2. Identify and demonstrate methods of emergency medical care for internal and external bleeding.

3. Explain the relationship between BSI and bleeding, and identify the measures that must be taken by the EMT-B for self-protection and patient protection.

4. Identify the importance of airway management for the trauma patient.

5. Identify the relationship between mechanism of injury and causes of internal bleeding.

6. Identify the signs and symptoms of shock and describe the appropriate management for internal and external bleeding.

7. State the principles of treatment for the patient with signs and symptoms of shock.

INTRODUCTION

This chapter covers the normal structure and function of the circulatory system and the failure of the circulatory system to function effectively. All body systems are dependent upon an adequate supply of well-oxygenated blood. Failure of the circulatory system may rapidly lead to severe illness, permanent injury, and death.

The EMT must be aware of the critical need for oxygen and adequate circulation in the human body. He or she must be able to identify rapidly the signs and symptoms of poor perfusion, and to properly manage these life-threatening conditions.

This chapter describes the effect of significant trauma on the circulatory system. It relates the signs and symptoms of inadequate circulation, along with an orientation to the skills needed to manage shock properly.

REVIEW QUESTIONS

1. The respiratory and circulatory systems are interrelated and the loss of normal function in one has a profoundly negative effect on the function of the other. (C 5-1.1)

   a. true
   b. false

2. The heart is located in the center of the chest, under the breastbone. In the adult, it is about the size of: (C 5-1.1)

   a. a clenched fist
   b. the jaw
   c. two clenched fists
   d. an ear

3. Which chambers of the heart are the largest and have the thickest walls? (C 5-1.1)

   a. veins
   b. atria
   c. ventricles
   d. arterioles

4. How many chambers are in the normal human heart? (C 5-1.1)

   a. 6
   b. 4
   c. 3
   d. 2

5. The upper chambers of the heart are the: (C 5-1.1)

   a. atria
   b. arteries
   c. arterioles
   d. aorta

6. The lower chambers of the heart are the: (C 5-1.1)

   a. venules
   b. ventricles
   c. vena cava
   d. vessels

7. The function of the heart is to pump blood through the vessels of the body to all areas that need it. (C 5-1.1)

   a. true
   b. false

8. The right atrium receives blood from the: (C 5-1.1)

   a. body
   b. lungs
   c. right ventricle
   d. pulmonary artery

9. The left atrium receives blood from the: (C 5-1.1)

   a. body
   b. lungs
   c. left ventricle
   d. aorta

10. The right ventricle receives blood from the: (C 5-1.1)

   a. right atrium and pumps it into the lungs
   b. left atrium and pumps it out to the body
   c. right atrium and pumps it into the body
   d. left atrium and pumps it out to the lungs

11. The left ventricle receives blood from the: (C 5-1.1)

   a. right ventricle and pumps it out to the lungs
   b. left atrium and pumps it out to the body
   c. right atrium and pumps it out to the body
   d. left atrium and pumps it out to the lungs

12. The flow of blood from the heart to the lungs and back to the heart is called: (C 5-1.1)

   a. hepatic perfusion
   b. systemic circulation
   c. pulmonary circulation
   d. renal circulation

13. The flow of blood from the heart through the body and back to the heart is called: (C 5-1.1)

   a. hepatic perfusion
   b. systemic circulation
   c. cystic circulation
   d. renal circulation

14. The valve that separates the right atrium from the right ventricle is the: (C 5-1.1)

   a. bicuspid
   b. mitral
   c. semilunar
   d. tricuspid

15. The valve that separates the left atrium from the left ventricle is the: (C 5-1.1)

   a. bicuspid
   b. lunar
   c. semilunar
   d. tricuspid

16. The ventricles are separated from the blood vessels by the: (C 5-1.1)
    a. mitral valves
    b. semilunar valves
    c. tricuspid valves
    d. lunar valves

17. Capillaries surround cells and provide oxygen and nutrients to the cells and remove waste products from the cells. (C 5-1.1)
    a. true
    b. false

18. The pulmonary arteries, located between the right ventricle and the lungs, are the only arteries that normally carry oxygen-rich blood. (C 5-1.1)
    a. true
    b. false

19. Red blood cells: (C 5-1.1)
    a. fight infection
    b. contain hemoglobin
    c. cause coagulation
    d. produce white blood cells

20. The human body is: (C 5-1.1)
    a. 60% water
    b. 80% water
    c. 75% water
    d. 20% water

21. The average adult blood volume is approximately: (C 5-1.6)
    a. 3,000 ml
    b. 5,000 ml
    c. 7,500 ml
    d. 500 ml

22. The total blood volume for a 1-year-old infant is approximately: (C 5-1.6)
    a. 2,000 ml
    b. 1,200 ml
    c. 800 ml
    d. 400 ml

23. Heart muscle is unique in that it generates electrical impulses on its own. (C 5-1.1)
    a. true
    b. false

24. Systolic pressure represents the: (C 5-1.1)
    a. second reading of the blood pressure
    b. first reading of the blood pressure
    c. blood pressure when the heart is relaxed
    d. venous blood pressure

25. Which of the following are good sites to palpate a pulse? (C 5-1.1)

    a. radial artery, brachial artery, femoral artery, carotid artery
    b. radial artery, pulmonary artery, femoral artery, carotid artery
    c. renal artery, pulmonary artery, femoral artery, carotid artery
    d. radial artery, brachial artery, hepatic artery, carotid artery

26. The apex of the heart points: (C 5-1.1)

    a. to the left
    b. to the right
    c. upward
    d. downward

27. Which of the following is/are primary causes of shock in the human body: (C 5-1.1)

    a. pump failure
    b. container failure
    c. volume failure
    d. all of the above

28. Hemorrhagic shock results from loss of blood volume. (C 5-1.9)

    a. true
    b. false

29. Neurogenic shock results from: (C 5-1.1)

    a. vasodilation
    b. hypovolemia
    c. vasoconstriction
    d. hypervolemia

30. During shock, the body attempts to survive by moving blood to the: (C 5-1.2)

    a. abdomen and heart from the legs, arms, lungs, and brain
    b. legs and lungs from the heart, abdomen, and brain
    c. heart and lungs from the legs, arms, and abdomen
    d. abdomen and brain from the heart, lungs, legs, and arms

31. Signs of an arterial bleed include: (C 5-1.2)

    a. oozing dark blood
    b. spurting bright red blood
    c. spurting dark blood
    d. all of the above

32. What is usually considered to be a severe sudden loss of blood in an adult? (C 5-1.2)

    a. 1000 cc
    b. 100 cc
    c. 250 cc
    d. 600 cc

33. Internal blood loss can be easily identified by an EMT. (C 5-1.7)

    a. true
    b. false

34. Signs of shock include: (C 5-1.9)

    a. rapid and weak pulse, pale skin
    b. cold and clammy skin, cyanosis
    c. increased respiratory rate, decreased level of consciousness
    d. all of the above

35. The rate of respiration, the color, temperature, and condition of the skin, and the depth of respiration should be evaluated: (C 5-1.10 and A 5-1.11)

    a. only in the ambulance
    b. only at the scene
    c. only during transport
    d. continuously

36. The proper location to check pulses for infants and small children is the: (C 5-1.9)

    a. brachial artery
    b. carotid artery
    c. posterior tibial artery
    d. radial artery

37. Normally, capillary refilling occurs in: (C 5-1.9)

    a. between 3 and 4 seconds
    b. greater than 2 seconds
    c. 2 seconds or less
    d. 3 seconds

38. A B/P of less than 90 mm Hg in the adult patient may be an indication that the patient is in crisis and unable to adequately perfuse their system. (C 5-1.9)

    a. true
    b. false

39. The most common site to palpate a B/P is the: (C 5-1.8)

    a. carotid artery
    b. brachial artery
    c. radial artery
    d. femoral artery

40. What is typically considered to be a severe sudden loss of blood in a child? (C 5-1.2)

    a. 50 cc
    b. 100 cc
    c. 250 cc
    d. 500 cc

41. Symptoms of shock include: (C 5-1.9)

    a. mental confusion, feeling of weakness
    b. feeling of impending doom, nausea
    c. vomiting, headache, thirst
    d. all of the above

42. The initial steps for management of shock include: (C 5-1.5)

    a. establishing and maintaining a patent airway
    b. administering high-flow oxygen and bleeding control
    c. managing hypotension and immediate transport
    d. all of the above

43. The trauma patient that is conscious and breathing on his or her own should be provided oxygen with a: (C 5-1.5)

    a. nonrebreather oxygen mask at 15 L/min flow
    b. nonrebreather oxygen mask at 5 L/min flow
    c. BVM at 15 L/min flow
    d. nasal cannula at 5 L/min flow

44. Any patient who is not breathing adequately on his or her own should receive support ventilations with a: (C 5-1.5)

    a. nonrebreather oxygen mask at 15 L/min flow
    b. nonrebreather oxygen mask at 5 L/min flow
    c. BVM at 15 L/min flow
    d. nasal cannula at 5 L/min flow

45. Any patient who demonstrates signs and symptoms of hypoperfusion should receive supplemental high-flow oxygen. (C 5-1.5)

    a. true
    b. false

46. A dressing should be placed over every visible wound to protect it from further injury and to prevent further contamination. (C 5-1.4)

    a. true
    b. false

47. If the dressing becomes saturated with blood: (C 5-1.3)

    a. nothing else can control the bleeding
    b. it should be replaced with a new dressing
    c. a new dressing should be placed on top of it
    d. a tourniquet should be applied

48. When bleeding is evident in an extremity, lowering the extremity may work to slow blood flow to the area and therefore, reduce the amount of blood lost. (C 5-1.3)

    a. true
    b. false

49. Pulse-point pressure should be used to control bleeding when: (C 5-1.3)

    a. direct pressure and/or elevation has not been effective
    b. when there is venous bleeding
    c. when there is capillary bleeding
    d. all of the above

50. What is generally considered to be a severe sudden loss of blood in an infant? (C 5-1.2)

    a. 50 cc
    b. 150 cc
    c. 15 cc
    d. 5 cc

51. The use of a tourniquet is: (C 5-1.3)

   a. the best method to control a venous bleed
   b. a last resort treatment for control of bleeding
   c. always used to control bleeding from an amputation
   d. only used for children

52. A patient that shows signs and symptoms of shock: (A 5-1.11)

   a. is not a high priority patient
   b. should be immediately transported
   c. should be allowed to drink water
   d. will have extremely high blood pressure

53. The ideal method of controlling hypotension for the patient in hypovolemic shock is to: (C 5-1.10)

   a. place the patient in left lateral recumbent position
   b. give glucose by mouth
   c. replace the lost blood volume
   d. give fluid by mouth

54. The delivery of fluids by mouth is a very effective method of fluid replacement when conscious patients, in severe shock, feel thirsty. (C 5-1.9)

   a. true
   b. false

55. Even though the Trendelenburg position uses gravity to assist in core perfusion, it increases pressure on the diaphragm and moves the abdominal organs against the diaphragm, making respirations more labored and difficult for the patient in crisis. (C 5-1.5)

   a. true
   b. false

56. Indications for the use of the Pneumatic Antishock Garment (PASG) include: (C 5-1.8)

   a. severe hypertension
   b. profound low blood pressure
   c. pulmonary edema
   d. all of the above

57. Which of the following are contraindications for the use of the PASG? (C 5-1.8)

   a. objects impaled in a site that would be covered
   b. the last 3 months of pregnancy
   c. pulmonary edema
   d. all of the above

58. Medical control is responsible, either directly or indirectly, for selection of the most appropriate treatment facilities for patients. (A 5-1.11)

   a. true
   b. false

59. Steps for managing shock include which of the following? (C 5-1.10)

    a. establishing a patent airway
    b. administering low-flow oxygen
    c. giving oral glucose
    d. giving fluids by mouth

60. The cardinal sign of shock is: (C 5-1.9)

    a. hypertension
    b. hypoperfusion
    c. hypotension
    d. perfusion

61. Metabolism that occurs in the presence of oxygen is best described as: (C 5-1.9)

    a. acidic
    b. aerobic
    c. anaerobic
    d. apneic

Scenario

Read each scenario. Write the answers to the corresponding questions in the space provided.

SCENARIO #1:

You and your paramedic partner have been called to the scene of a shooting incident. When you arrive at the scene, law enforcement officers are present and the patient is lying supine on the ground beside the door steps. The female involved in the incident reports that the patient was running out of the front door when he was shot by a distraught male who was also on the scene.

Upon assessment of the patient, you note no blood on the ground around the patient. An entrance wound is visible in the right forearm and you note that there is no bleeding from this wound. There are entrance and exit wounds found on the upper lateral thigh and an entrance wound in the right upper back.

A carotid pulse is present, but radial pulses are absent. The patient is unresponsive. His skin is pale and clammy. Capillary fill time is greater than 4 seconds. The respiratory rate is 30 breaths/min and shallow. Blood pressure en route to the hospital is noted to be 60/40.

1. What are the scene safety considerations?

2. When should this patient be transported?

continued

3 Describe at least five interventions that should be performed at the scene.

_____

_____

_____

_____

4 Describe at least three interventions that should be performed during transport.

_____

_____

_____

_____

CHAPTER 31 ANSWERS TO REVIEW QUESTIONS

1.	a	14.	d	27.	d	40.	d	53.	c
2.	a	15.	a	28.	a	41.	d	54.	b
3.	c	16.	b	29.	a	42.	d	55.	a
4.	b	17.	a	30.	c	43.	a	56.	b
5.	a	18.	b	31.	b	44.	c	57.	d
6.	b	19.	b	32.	a	45.	a	58.	a
7.	a	20.	a	33.	b	46.	a	59.	a
8.	a	21.	b	34.	d	47.	c	60.	b
9.	b	22.	c	35.	d	48.	b	61.	b
10.	a	23.	a	36.	a	49.	a		
11.	b	24.	b	37.	c	50.	b		
12.	c	25.	a	38.	a	51.	b		
13.	b	26.	d	39.	c	52.	b		

SCENARIO SOLUTIONS

Scenario #1:

1. Scene safety considerations are that the incident involves weapons, therefore the law enforcement officers must be in control of the scene. Personal safety must be the primary concern for the EMT. Body substance isolation precautions should be taken.
2. The patient should be transported as soon as possible.
3. Interventions that should be performed are as follows:
   a. Assist ventilations with a bag-valve-mask attached to high-flow oxygen.
   b. Any open wounds to the chest should be covered with an occlusive dressing.
   c. The PASG should be applied according to local protocols.
   d. Complete spinal packaging.

4. Interventions that should be performed during transport are as follows:
   a. Assist ventilations with a BVM attached to high-flow oxygen.
   b. Look for wounds that may have been missed and initiate wound management.
   c. Reassess patient's vital signs frequently.
   d. Communicate with medical control.

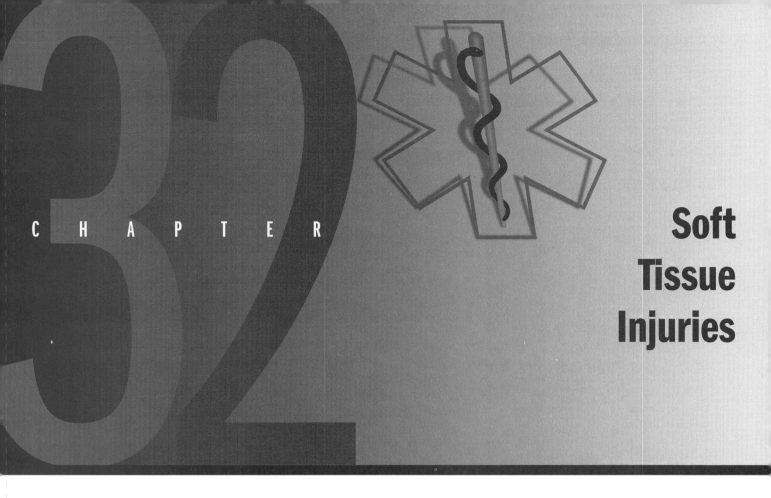

Soft Tissue Injuries

Reading Assignment: Chapter 32, pgs. 577–592

OBJECTIVES

1. Describe the anatomy and physiology of the skin.

2. List the types and describe the emergency medical care for closed and open soft tissue injuries.

3. Describe and contrast the emergency medical care considerations for a penetrating chest injury and an open abdominal wound.

4. Describe the purpose and function of dressings and bandages, and outline the steps in the application of a pressure dressing.

5. Describe the effects of improperly applied dressings, splints, and tourniquets.

6. Describe the emergency medical care of a patient with an impaled object or a traumatic amputation.

INTRODUCTION

Soft tissue injuries are among the most common injuries that the EMT will encounter. This chapter deals with soft tissue injuries, ranging from simple bruises to large wounds. Soft tissue injuries are often found with broken bones.

The treatment of the soft tissue wounds may directly affect the amount and type of damage that is received by the underlying organs and may also affect recovery time. This chapter emphasizes bleeding control, prevention of other injuries, and reducing contamination.

REVIEW QUESTIONS

Please circle one correct answer for each question.

1. The largest organ of the body is the: (C 5-2.1)
   a. heart
   b. liver
   c. skin
   d. kidney

2. What are the layers of the skin? (C 5-2.2)
   a. the epidermis, dermis, and subcutaneous tissue
   b. the outer dermis, dermis, and subcutaneous tissue
   c. the epidermis, dermis, and muscle tissue
   d. the middermis, dermis, and subcutaneous tissue

3. What is the outermost layer of the skin? (C 5-2.2)
   a. peridermis
   b. subcutaneous tissue
   c. the epidermis
   d. the dermis

4. The dermis contains: (C 5-2.2)
   a. blood vessels and lymphatic vessels
   b. nerve endings and hair follicles
   c. sweat glands and sebaceous glands
   d. all of the above

5. The deepest layer of the skin, the subcutaneous tissue, is composed of: (C 5-2.2)
   a. fatty tissue
   b. fibrous tissue
   c. elastic tissue
   d. all of the above

6. Which of the following are functions of the skin: (C 5-2.1)
   a. protection from invading microorganisms
   b. prevention of fluid loss
   c. maintenance of normal body temperature
   d. all of the above

7. A method to determine the size of the skin area that may be damaged by burns or abrasions is the: (C 5-2.6)
   a. rule of nines
   b. EMS rule
   c. rule of sixes
   d. rule of eights

8. The palm of the patient's hand is equal to about: (C 5-2.6)

   a. 3% body surface area
   b. 4% body surface area
   c. 1% body surface area
   d. 6% body surface area

9. Closed soft tissue injuries occur when the skin is broken. (C 5-2.4)

   a. true
   b. false

10. Which of the following is not a closed soft tissue injury? (C 5-2.4)

    a. contusion
    b. avulsion
    c. hematoma
    d. crush injury

11. Which of the following are open soft tissue injuries? (C 5-2.6)

    a. abrasions, lacerations
    b. avulsions, penetrating wounds
    c. puncture wounds, amputations
    d. all of the above

12. Contusions are commonly called: (C 5-2.4)

    a. lacerations
    b. bruises
    c. abrasions
    d. avulsions

13. In severe injuries the hematoma may contain one or more liters of blood. This may lead to hypotension and shock. (C 5-2.4)

    a. true
    b. false

14. When part of the body is caught between two compressing surfaces, a _____ injury results. (C 5-2.4)

    a. penetrating
    b. crush
    c. push
    d. shear

15. Forceful impact with a sharp object can produce a break in the skin of varying depth. This type of injury is called a(n): (C 5-2.6)

    a. abrasion
    b. crush
    c. laceration
    d. contusion

16. Flaps of skin or tissue may be torn loose or pulled completely off. This kind of injury is called a(n): (C 5-2.6)

    a. avulsion
    b. amputation
    c. laceration
    d. contusion

17. Penetrating wounds are caused by sharp, pointed objects that puncture the skin. The most common penetrating injuries are caused by: (C 5-2.6)

   a. gunshots
   b. knife stabs
   c. baseball bats
   d. a and b

18. Exit wounds may be present with gunshot wounds. It is important to: (C 5-2.7 and C 5-2.8)

   a. perform a careful secondary survey
   b. identify all injuries
   c. guard against focusing on a single penetrating injury
   d. all of the above

19. Increasing the pressure outside the vessel decreases the amount of blood that leaks out of the hole. The best method to accomplish this goal is: (C 5-2.7)

   a. direct pressure
   b. tourniquet
   c. wound irrigation
   d. indirect pressure

20. Hemorrhage from certain injuries can be massive, with up to 1 or 2 L of blood being lost. Examples of these injuries include all of the following **except:** (C 5-2.4)

   a. liver lacerations
   b. pelvic fractures
   c. femur fractures
   d. radial fractures

21. Most closed soft tissue injuries do not require treatment in the field by the EMT. (C 5-2.5)

   a. true
   b. false

22. Proper management of open soft tissue injuries includes which of the following? (C 5-2.7)

   a. application of a sterile dressing
   b. immediate control of severe external hemorrhage
   c. cover the patient
   d. all of the above

23. Why should wet dressings not be applied to a large open soft tissue injury? (C 5-2.5)

   a. wet dressings cause evaporative heat loss
   b. wet dressings cause heat retention
   c. wet dressings cause severe blood clots
   d. wet dressings promote patient comfort

24. An EMT must use BSI measures any time soft tissue injuries are present because of the accompanying blood. (C 5-2.3)

   a. true
   b. false

25. Proper management for eviscerations includes: (C 5-2.9)

   a. pushing the organ back into the body
   b. placing a dry, sterile dressing over the injury
   ⓒ placing a moist dressing over the injury
   d. using paper towels as a dressing

26. What action(s) should be taken when caring for a patient with an amputation or avulsion? (C 5-2.27)

   a. locate the detached body part
   b. package the body part in a plastic bag
   c. transport the body part with the patient
   ⓓ all of the above

27. Treatment modalities common to both chest and abdominal injuries include all of the following **except:** (C 5-2.10)

   ⓐ sterile occlusive dressing
   b. supplemental oxygen
   c. assessment of airway, breathing, and circulation
   d. expeditious transport to the hospital

28. Which of the following are goals of dressings and bandages? (C 5-2.21 and C 5-2.22)

   a. prevention of further contamination
   b. protection from additional injury
   c. decreased fluid loss from the disrupted skin
   ⓓ all of the above

29. Air-tight (occlusive) dressings should be used for open chest wounds to prevent air from being sucked into the chest cavity. (C 5-2.8)

   ⓐ true
   b. false

30. Impaled objects should only be removed prior to arrival in the hospital when the object interferes with chest compressions, establishment of an airway, or the transport of the patient. (C 5-2.26)

   ⓐ true
   b. false

31. Impaled objects can be properly managed by: (C 5-2.26)

   a. removal at the scene
   ⓑ stabilization with a bulky dressing
   c. pushing the object out of the wound
   d. irrigating the object with saline

32. Amputated body parts should be kept cool by soaking them in saline and placing them directly on ice. (C 5-2.27)

   a. true
   ⓑ false

33. Which of the following is true concerning open wounds to the neck? (C 5-2.7)

   a. severe hemorrhage is possible
   b. an air embolism is possible
   c. a sterile occlusive dressing should be applied
   ⓓ all of the above

34. When applying a pressure dressing, it should be placed tightly enough to insure that blood flow distal to the wound is occluded. (C 5-2.23)

    a. true
    b. false

35. Any patient with a knife wound to the chest and difficulty breathing should be assumed to have an open chest wound until evaluated by a physician. (C 5-2.24)

    a. true
    b. false

36. The mainstay treatment of a patient with chemical burns to the eyes is: (C 5-2.28)

    a. dressings and bandages to the injured eye only
    b. copious irrigation
    c. dressings applied over both eyes
    d. gauze pads soaked with saline

37. When dealing with victims of electrical burns, the primary concern for the EMT is: (C 5-2.29)

    a. personal safety
    b. patient safety
    c. crew safety
    d. bystander safety

38. Improperly applied dressings, splints, and tourniquets can lead to: (C 5-2.25)

    a. further damage to injured areas
    b. continued contamination
    c. possible limb loss from compromised blood flow
    d. all of the above

Scenario

Read each scenario. Write the answers to the corresponding questions in the space provided.

SCENARIO #1:

Today is the fourth of July. You and your partner are called to a residence where a hysterical woman meets you in the driveway. She tells you that your patient is a 10-year-old male who was attending her son's birthday party. The child had been riding a bicycle when he lost control of the bike and crashed into the plate glass window of her patio.

You find the child lying on the patio and you immediately notice that there is massive bleeding from the face, neck and left arm. The boy complains of difficulty breathing. There is a wound on the left side of his neck and a small open wound to the chest. He complains of pain in his left arm.

continued

1. What is the first step you should take?

_____

_____

_____

2. In assessing and managing the face and neck injuries, name at least four treatment considerations.

_____

_____

_____

_____

CHAPTER 32 ANSWERS TO REVIEW QUESTIONS

1. c	9. b	17. d	25. c
2. a	10. b	18. d	26. d
3. c	11. d	19. a	27. a
4. d	12. b	20. d	28. d
5. d	13. a	21. a	29. a
6. d	14. b	22. d	30. a
7. a	15. c	23. a	31. b
8. c	16. a	24. a	32. b
			33. d
			34. b
			35. a
			36. b
			37. a
			38. d

SCENARIO SOLUTIONS

Scenario #1

1. After implementing BSI precautions, your first step would be to assess and clear the airway, while gaining control of the cervical spine. Suction the airway as needed.

2. Treatment considerations are as follows:

- The bleeding wounds should be assessed for the severity of hemorrhage and the amount of blood already lost.
- A sterile dressing with direct pressure should be applied to the facial injuries.
- An occlusive dressing may be needed to treat the neck injury adequately in order to control bleeding and to avoid air entering the large vessels of the neck.
- The breathing problems may be caused by air inside the chest between the chest wall and lung (pneumothorax) and the patient has an open wound on his chest. The open chest wound should be assumed to penetrate into the thoracic cavity. It should be treated with an occlusive dressing.
- The extremity injuries are assessed and treated at the scene only if the patient is stable and does not require rapid transport to the hospital.
- The patient must be spinal packaged and rapidly transported to an appropriate hospital.

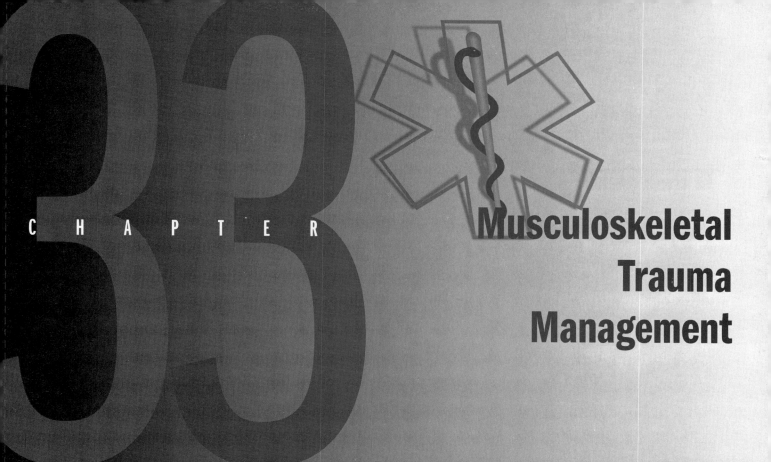

Musculoskeletal Trauma Management

Reading Assignment: Chapter 33, pgs. 593–613

OBJECTIVES

1. Describe the functions of the muscular system.

2. Describe the functions of the skeletal system.

3. List the major bones and groups of bones in the:
   a. Upper extremities
   b. Lower extremities

4. Define the signs and symptoms of a fracture, dislocation, and sprain.

5. Define splinting and describe the benefits and complications of splinting.

6. Describe the general principles of splinting.

7. Describe the treatment (besides splinting) of a fracture, dislocation, and sprain.

INTRODUCTION

Musculoskeletal injuries are commonly seen in EMS. This chapter presents a discussion of musculoskeletal injuries so that the EMT can gain a general perspective of musculoskeletal injuries and their care.

Field management of painful, swollen, deformed extremities is centered around the importance of proper immobilization of the injured limb. The injured limb is immobilized or stabilized so that the patient's pain is reduced and further injury is minimized.

REVIEW QUESTIONS

Please circle one correct answer for each question.

1. The medical term for a broken bone is a: (Chp. Obj. #4)

    a. fracture
    b. dislocation
    c. displacement
    d. sprain

2. A strain is also known as a: (Chp. Obj. #4)

    a. fracture
    b. muscle pull
    c. ligamentous
    d. sprain

3. Determining the mechanism of injury is important because this knowledge may help to determine the nature and the extent of the injury. (Chp. Obj. #4)

    a. true
    b. false

4. The major support of the upper skeletal extremity and its attachment to the body is achieved through muscles that originate on the rib cage and insert onto either the scapula or the humerus. (C 5-3.1 and C 5-3.2)

    a. true
    b. false

5. The bones of the upper extremities include all of the following **except:** (C 5-3.3)

    a. scapula
    b. clavicle
    c. femur
    d. humerus

6. A painful, swollen, deformed extremity, in which the skin integrity has been compromised is called a(n) _____ injury. (C 5-3.4)

    a. open
    b. closed
    c. vertical
    d. compromised

7. Adequate assessment of distal pulses, movement and sensation in painful, swollen, deformed extremities includes all of the following **except:** (C 5-3.8)

    a. check the pulses prior to splinting
    b. check the pulses after splinting
    c. check the pulse during splinting
    d. pulse checks after splinting are sufficient

8. If the determination has been made that the patient has a life-threatening injury, painful, swollen, deformed extremities can be splinted using an anatomical splint, such as a long spine board. (C 5-3.9)

   ⓐ true
   b. false

9. Crepitus: (Chp. Obj. #4)

   a. is a sound bones can make when they are broken
   b. is the feeling caused by grating of bone ends against each other
   c. can cause further damage, if improperly manipulated
   ⓓ both a and b

10. Bones of the lower extremities include all of the following **except:** (C 5-3.3)

    a. pelvis
    b. femur
    ⓒ scapula
    d. tibia

11. If a painful, swollen, deformed extremity exists, it is the responsibility of the EMT to immobilize the extremity so that no further injury occurs to the patient. (A 5-3.10)

    ⓐ true
    b. false

12. The most common complications of painful, swollen, deformed extremities include all of the following **except:** (C 5-3.11)

    a. edema
    b. hemorrhage
    c. discoloration
    ⓓ proper alignment

13. The dislodging of a bone from its normal position in a joint is called a: (Chp. Obj. #4)

    ⓐ dislocation
    b. strain
    c. sprain
    d. abrasion

14. Signs and symptoms to look for when assessing a painful, swollen, deformed extremity include: (C 5-3.4)

    a. deformity, crepitus
    b. swelling, discoloration
    c. pain, loss of sensation or movement
    ⓓ all of the above

15. Complications of splinting may include all of the following **except:** (C 5-3.7)

    ⓐ external hemorrhage
    b. circulatory compromise
    c. muscle damage
    d. nerve damage

16. Injuries to muscles are more common than injuries to bones. (C 5-3.4)

a. true
b. false

17. It is not the responsibility of an EMT to differentiate between a muscle injury and a bone injury. (C 5-3.6)

a. true
b. false

18. A _____ is a soft tissue injury or muscle spasm that occurs around a joint anywhere in the musculature. (Chp. Obj. #4)

a. strain
b. sprain
c. laceration
d. bruise

19. Acute swelling of an extremity indicates: (C 5-3.4)

a. hemorrhage
b. inflammation
c. both a and b
d. neither a nor b

20. If no life threatening conditions are evident, the EMT should splint the patient's injury before moving him. (A 5-3.9)

a. true
b. false

21. Traction splints are indicated for: (C 5-3.6)

a. painful, swollen, deformed ankles
b. painful, swollen, deformed elbows
c. painful, swollen, deformed hips
d. painful, swollen, deformed midthigh areas

22. If a severe deformity exists or the distal extremity is cyanotic or lacks pulses, the EMT should align with gentle traction before splinting. (C 5-3.6)

a. true
b. false

23. The extremity should be supported while being splinted, thus splinting requires two people. (C 5-3.6)

a. true
b. false

24. Examples of long bone splints include padded long boards and ladder splints. These splints are used to treat deformities of the: (C 5-3.6)

a. humerus
b. radius
c. ulna
d. all of the above

25. Sling and swathe bandages are also called: (C 5-3.6)

   a. cravats
   b. triangle bandages
   c. a and b
   d. occlusive dressings

26. Painful, swollen, deformed extremities must be supported while being splinted. (C 5-3.6)

   a. true
   b. false

Scenario

Read each scenario. Write the answers to the corresponding questions in the space provided.

SCENARIO #1:

You and your partner have been dispatched to the scene where a 40-year-old male patient fell from a 20-ft, A-frame ladder to the concrete.

   Your patient responds to pain. Assessment reveals a midshaft thigh injury, a distal radius injury, and an open head injury.

1. List steps taken to prepare the patient for transport.

   _____

   _____

   _____

   _____

2. List interventions to be performed en route to the definitive care facility.

   _____

   _____

   _____

   _____

   _____

CHAPTER 33 ANSWERS TO REVIEW QUESTIONS

1. a	6. a	11. a	16. a	21. d
2. b	7. d	12. d	17. a	22. a
3. a	8. a	13. a	18. a	23. a
4. a	9. d	14. d	19. c	24. d
5. c	10. c	15. a	20. a	25. c
6. a	11. a	16. a	21. d	26. a

SCENARIO SOLUTIONS

Scenario #1:

1. Steps to prepare this patient for transport are as follows:
   a. Upon arrival at the scene, C-spine immobilization is indicated, since the patient fell.
   b. Assess ABCs.
   c. Continually assess his level of consciousness (LOC).
   d. Administer oxygen.
   e. Place patient on a long spine board. (Spinal packaging as per local protocol.)
   f. Consider PASG, as indicated per local protocol.
   g. Initiate immediate transport—concurrent with medical control —to the definitive care facility.
2. En route to the definitive care facility:
   a. Perform an ongoing assessment.
   b. Splint the extremities as indicated.
   c. Note capillary refill and color.
   d. Monitor and record vital signs.
   e. Assess pulses, movement and sensation after applying splint.
   f. Call the hospital to inform them of your patient's condition and time of arrival.

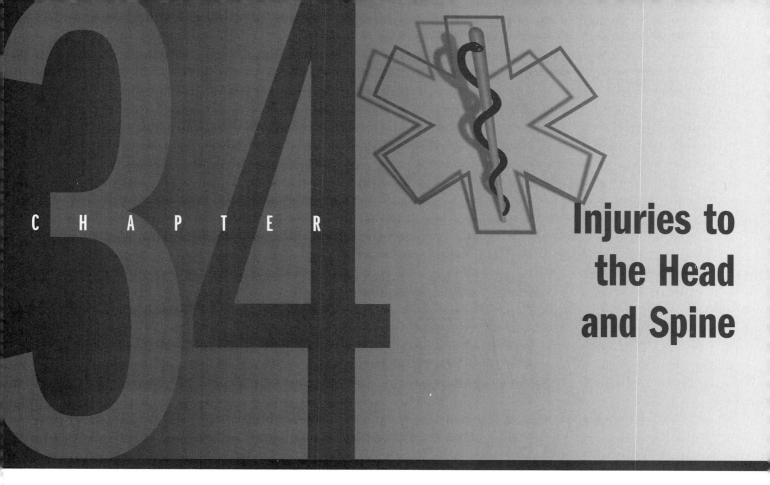

CHAPTER 34

Injuries to the Head and Spine

Reading Assignment: Chapter 34, pgs. 614–642

OBJECTIVES

1. State the components and functions of the structures of the head and spine.

2. Describe the relationship of mechanism of injury to potential injuries of the head and spine.

3. List the signs and symptoms of a potential head injury.

4. Discuss airway emergency medical care techniques for the patient with a suspected spine and/or head injury.

5. Describe how to stabilize the cervical spine.

6. Discuss indications for sizing and method for using a cervical spine immobilization device.

7. Describe how and when to secure a patient to a long and short spine board.

8. Identify when to use rapid extrication.

9. Discuss when and how to remove different types of helmets and the criteria that contribute to the decision to remove a helmet.

INTRODUCTION

This chapter presents the EMT student with information necessary to properly assess and manage head and spine injuries. The interventions included in this chapter could mean the difference between life and death or permanent disability for the patient who has head or spinal injuries.

EMTs are called upon to perform a diverse range of skills of which two of the most important are the ability to identify head and spinal injuries properly and the ability to immobilize the head and spine effectively. Patients who have an unstable spine could die or be permanently harmed if these injuries are treated improperly in the field.

REVIEW QUESTIONS

Please circle one correct answer for each question.

1. Altered mental status is the single most important sign of a head injury. (Chp. Obj. #3)

   (a) true
   b. false

2. Regarding the head-injured patient, all of the following statements are true **except:** (Chp. Obj. #3)

   a. mental status must be evaluated critically and continually
   b. assessment information must be documented for legal reasons
   c. it is important to fully apprise the hospital staff of any change in the patient's condition
   (d) if the patient is ambulatory at the scene, spinal precautions are not needed

3. Mechanism of injury is essential information to obtain in the identification of injuries the patient may have sustained. (C 5-4.4)

   (a) true
   b. false

4. The head contains one of the most important organs of the body. This organ is the: (C 5-4.1)

   a. cranium
   (b) brain
   c. scalp
   d. meninges

5. The _____ is the outermost part of the head and contains numerous tissues, including the hair follicles, sweat glands, sebaceous glands, and many of the blood vessels and capillaries. (C 5-4.3)

   a. cranium
   b. brain
   (c) scalp
   d. meninges

6. Because the head is very vascular, the scalp tends to bleed freely. This bleeding can be easily controlled. (C 5-4.3)

   a. true
   (b) false

7. The most efficient method to handle scalp bleeding is: (Chp. Obj. #4)

   a. pressure points
   b. tourniquets
   c. direct pressure
   d. pressure dressings

8. The skull or cranium is comprised of all of the following bones **except:** (C 5-4.3)

   a. frontal
   b. occipital
   c. tibial
   d. temporal

9. These bones are joined by immobile interlocking joints called: (C 5-4.3)

   a. joints
   b. sutures
   c. openings
   d. foramen

10. Located at the base of the skull is an opening through which the brain stem and the spinal cord pass. This opening is called the: (C 5-4.3)

    a. foramen magnum
    b. calcaneus
    c. circle of Willis
    d. orifice

11. Highly vascular membranes separate the cranium and the brain. These membranes include all of the following **except:** (C 5-4.1)

    a. dura mater
    b. arachnoid membrane
    c. pia mater
    d. tunica intima

12. The membranes referenced in Question #11 are collectively known as the: (C 5-4.1)

    a. meninges
    b. ventricles
    c. foramen
    d. brain tissues

13. Epidural hematoma is a condition in which blood leaks into the epidural space. (C 5-4.4)

    a. true
    b. false

14. In evaluating the mechanism of injury, a skilled EMT should do all of the following **except:** (C 5-4.4)

    a. properly use bystanders as a source of information
    b. evaluate the evidence on the scene and look at the vehicle
    c. rely solely on information provided by the patient
    d. examine entrance and exit wounds

15. The nervous system is divided into two parts, the central nervous system and the: (C 5-4.1)

    a. core nervous system
    b. superficial nervous system
    c. peripheral nervous system
    d. marginal nervous system

16. The brain is divided into the: (C 5-4.1)

    a. cerebrum
    b. cerebellum
    c. brain stem
    d. all of the above

17. The medulla is located in the brain stem and is responsible for vital functions of the body such as: (C 5-4.2)

    a. heart rate
    b. respiratory rate
    c. blood pressure
    d. all of the above

18. Cerebrospinal fluid (CSF) is produced in the brain and is found within the: (C 5-4.2)

    a. subarachnoid space
    b. dural space
    c. potential space
    d. foramenal space

19. Cerebrospinal fluid serves as a: (C 5-4.2)

    a. shock absorber
    b. mechanism for leakage to the outside
    c. deterrent to bacteria entering the brain
    d. place for production of red blood cells

20. Open head injuries have three complications that are not associated with closed head injuries. These complications include all of the following **except:** (C 5-4.2)

    a. potential for developing increased intracranial pressure
    b. leakage of CSF outside of the body
    c. possible bacterial contamination of the brain through the injury
    d. herniation of the brain through the defect in the skull

21. "Increased intracranial pressure" is the increase of pressure inside the skull caused by fluid accumulation. (Chp. Obj. #3)

    a. true
    b. false

22. All of the following are signs known as Cushing's triad **except:** (Chp. Obj. #3)

    a. an increase in blood pressure
    b. a change in respiratory effort
    c. an increase in pulse rate
    d. decrease in pulse rate

23. Head trauma is the leading cause of traumatic death, and the majority of these injuries result from motor vehicle crashes. (C 5-4.4)

    a. true
    b. false

24. Periorbital ecchymosis (black eye) is caused by blood accumulating in the tissue around the eye. This condition is called: (Chp. Obj. #3)

    a. Kernig's sign
    b. Battle's sign
    c. raccoon's eyes
    d. Horner's sign

25. Level of consciousness is an indirect measurement of the cerebral oxygenation. (C 5-4.2)

    a. true
    b. false

26. Level of consciousness is described by using the acronym: (C 5-4.7)

    a. AVPU
    b. SAMPLE
    c. PQRST
    d. APUV

27. The spinal column is composed of 33 bones called: (C 5-4.3)

    a. disc
    b. vertebrae
    c. meninges
    d. phalanges

28. The 33 bones that comprise the spinal column are divided into: (C 5-4.3)

    a. 7 cervical, 12 thoracic
    b. 5 lumbar, 5 sacral
    c. 4 coccyx vertebrae
    d. all of the above

29. Determining the mechanism of injury is one of the crucial responsibilities of an EMT. An EMT must maintain a high index of suspicion for head and spinal injuries when any of the following has occurred **except:** (C 5-4.4)

    a. motor vehicle crashes (pedestrian vs. vehicle crash)
    b. falls, blunt trauma
    c. motorcycle or bicycle crashes
    d. distal extremity lacerations

30. If the EMT suspects that the patient has spinal trauma, he or she should initiate spinal precautions. Undertreatment may result in paraplegia (paralysis from the waist down) or quadriplegia (paralysis from the neck down). (C 5-4.5)

    a. true
    b. false

31. Signs and symptoms associated with spinal injuries include all of the following **except:** (C 5-4.6)

    a. quadriplegia
    b. paraplegia
    c. hypoglycemia
    d. point tenderness and pain

32. The patient's ability to walk should not alter your suspicion regarding the possibility of spinal injuries. (C 5-4.6)

    a. true
    b. false

33. The appropriate time to control the spine is: (C 5-4.9)

    a. prior to assessing the airway
    b. after assessing the airway
    c. during transportation to the hospital
    d. after the application of the PASG

34. Spinal immobilization should be maintained until spinal injury has been completely ruled out by the EMT. (C 5-4.10)

    a. true
    b. false

35. The EMT must put the patient's head in a _____ inline position to open the airway; this is an opportune time to establish control of the spine. (C 5-4.8 and C 5-4.11)

    a. flexed
    b. neutral
    c. hyperextended
    d. pronate

36. To establish a patent airway on an unresponsive patient who has a suspected spinal injury, the EMT should use the: (C 5-4.8)

    a. head-tilt chin-lift technique
    b. modified jaw-thrust
    c. head-tilt neck-lift technique
    d. jaw-thrust lift with head tilt

37. An improperly fitting immobilization device will do more harm than good. (C 5-4.12)

    a. true
    b. false

38. Responsibilities of the EMT who is maintaining inline immobilization of the spine include all of the following **except:** (C 5-4.12)

    a. maintaining constant, inline control of the spine
    b. maintaining C-spine control only when logrolling the patient
    c. continual airway assessment
    d. maintaining this duty until the patient is immobilized to the long board

39. When the patient is ready to be placed on the long spine board: (C 5-4.14)

   a. one EMT maintains manual inline immobilization
   b. the other EMT positions the board next to the patient
   c. the EMT at the patient's head directs the movement of the patient
   d. all of the above

40. Short back boards may be used: (C 5-4.15)

   a. to immobilize seated, noncritical patients with suspected spinal injuries
   b. as a long spine board for a pediatric patient
   c. both a and b
   d. neither a nor b

41. Initial steps used in applying the short back board include: (C 5-4.16)

   a. the first EMT initiates manual spinal immobilization and performs the initial survey
   b. the second EMT performs the ongoing survey and prepares to apply the cervical collar and the short spine board
   c. the second EMT positions the device behind patient
   d. all of the above

42. During application of the short back board, the EMT should continue an ongoing assessment, paying close attention to assessing pulse, movement, and sensation in all extremities. (C 5-4.16)

   a. true
   b. false

43. Indications for rapid extrication of the patient include all of the following **except:** (C 5-4.17)

   a. an unsafe scene
   b. a patient's life threatening condition requires immediate transport to the appropriate facility
   c. when a family member or friend prevents the EMT from caring for a patient
   d. when the police are present, in control of the scene and the patient is stable

44. When considering the steps of rapid extrication, the EMT should remember that it is important to check ABC's prior to extrication. (C 5-4.18)

   a. true
   b. false

45. Sports helmets typically open in the: (C 5-4.22)

   a. left side
   b. back
   c. front
   d. right side

46. Two types of helmets most likely to be seen in the prehospital environment are the sports helmet and the: (C 5-4.21)

    a. motorcycle helmet
    b. skater's helmet
    c. flight helmet
    d. military helmet

47. Considerations regarding whether the helmet should be removed or left in place include all of the following **except:** (C 5-4.19 and C 5-4.20)

    a. fit of the helmet and patient's movement within the helmet
    b. impending airway or breathing problem
    c. transport time to definitive care
    d. proper spinal immobilization must be provided

48. When considering methods for helmet removal, the EMT should remember that a minimum of ___ EMTs should participate in the technique: (C 5-4.23 and C 5-4.24)

    a. 1
    b. 2
    c. 3
    d. 4

49. Proper spinal immobilization must be maintained whether the helmet is left in place or removed. (C 5-4.25 and C 5-4.26)

    a. true
    b. false

50. Small children and infants not found in a car seat can be immobilized on a short spine board, providing the legs do not hang over the edge. (C 5-4.15)

    a. true
    b. false

Scenario

Read each scenario. Write the answers to the corresponding questions in the space provided.

SCENARIO #1:

At 1800 hours on a hot summer afternoon, you and your crew are called to a scene where a 6-year-old female has fallen from the back of a moving vehicle. Upon arrival at the scene, you find the child combative and responsive only to painful stimuli. The child is exhibiting signs of increased intracranial pressure and Battle's sign is present. You note blood on the asphalt beneath the patient's head. Patient's respirations are labored and rapid.

Looking at the vehicle, you determine the fall was approximately 3 ft. Family members state that the child was immediately "knocked unconscious." Obvious head trauma is noted.

continued

1. What are your initial management considerations?

    _____

    _____

    _____

    _____

2. What is your transport decision?

    _____

    _____

    _____

    _____

3. What are the packaging considerations as you manage this situation?

    _____

    _____

    _____

    _____

4. Name at least four interventions to be performed en route to the definitive care facility.

    _____

    _____

    _____

    _____

    _____

CHAPTER 34 ANSWERS TO REVIEW QUESTIONS

1. a	**11.** d	**21.** a	**31.** c	**41.** d
2. d	**12.** a	**22.** c	**32.** a	**42.** a
3. a	**13.** a	**23.** a	**33.** a	**43.** d
4. b	**14.** c	**24.** c	**34.** b	**44.** a
5. c	**15.** c	**25.** a	**35.** b	**45.** c
6. b	**16.** d	**26.** a	**36.** b	**46.** a
7. c	**17.** d	**27.** b	**37.** a	**47.** c
8. c	**18.** a	**28.** d	**38.** b	**48.** b
9. b	**19.** a	**29.** d	**39.** d	**49.** a
10. a	**20.** a	**30.** a	**40.** c	**50.** a

SCENARIO SOLUTIONS

Scenario #1

1. Initial management considerations include:

- C-spine immobilization
- Airway
- Breathing
- Circulation

2. Your transport decision should be to "load and go," based on the patient's critical condition, mechanism of injury, and compromise of mental status.

3. Due to the mechanism of injury, the patient requires full spinal immobilization on an emergent basis. Based on patient size, a short back board may be the immobilization device of choice. Padding behind the shoulders should be considered to maintain inline stabilization properly.

4. Interventions to be performed en route include:

    - Airway management
    - Oxygen administration
    - Wound management
    - Continue evaluation of LOC
    - Carefully observe vital sign changes
    - Neuro checks to include evaluation of pulse, motor and sensory. Pupils should be closely evaluated

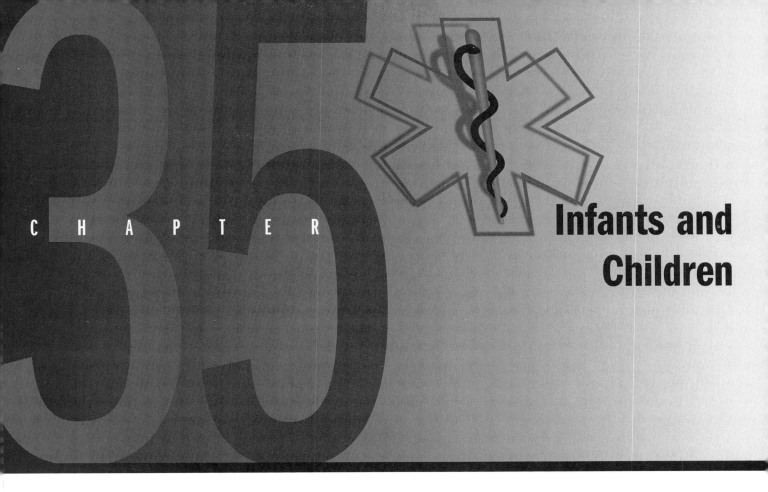

CHAPTER 35

Infants and Children

Reading Assignment: Chapter 35, pgs. 643–682

OBJECTIVES

1. Identify approach strategies for different pediatric developmental stages.

2. Recognize signs and symptoms of increased respiratory effort in the infant or child.

3. Recognize signs and symptoms of shock in the infant or child.

4. List three techniques to accomplish effective BVM ventilation in the infant or child.

5. List three characteristics of the following diseases:
   - Croup
   - Epiglottitis
   - Asthma (reactive airways disease)
   - Bronchiolitis

6. Describe the treatment of an infant or child in status epilepticus.

7. Identify signs and symptoms of an infant or child with
   - Meningitis
   - Dehydration

8. List the causes of pediatric injuries in order of most to least common.

9. List three activities that may cause spinal trauma in the pediatric patient.

10. List three of the most common types of poisons in children.

11. List five risk factors for child maltreatment.

12. List five indicators of child abuse.

INTRODUCTION

Infant and child patients often cause anxiety for the prehospital care provider. These patients may present special demands for the EMT-B.

This chapter details the special factors involved, such as body size, developmental considerations and normal ranges of vital signs. It reviews techniques for BLS and discusses several medical and trauma emergencies, including assessment and treatment modalities.

REVIEW QUESTIONS

Please circle one correct answer for each question.

1. Which of the following techniques is NOT useful when treating a toddler? (C 6-1.1)

    a. Choose words carefully when explaining the child's injury to him or her.
    b. Let the child play with your stethoscope while getting a history from the parents.
    c. Remove the child from his or her mother to finish the physical examination.
    d. Tell the child in simple terms what you are going to do.

2. All of following are signs of increased respiratory effort in the infant or child **except:** (C 6-1.5)

    a. sternal retractions
    b. head bobbing
    c. nasal flaring
    d. bradypnea

3. A childhood disease, usually caused by a bacterial infection, that has a rapid onset and results in the child drooling while sitting in the "tripod" position is: (C 6-1.4)

    a. croup
    b. bronchiolitis
    c. epiglottitis
    d. asthma

4. The term "postictal" is associated with which of the following emergencies: (C 6-1.12)

    a. meningitis
    b. seizure
    c. head trauma
    d. dehydration

5. Major fears of the school-age child include all of the following **except:** (C 6-1.1)

    a. death
    b. loss of control
    c. strangers
    d. bodily injury and/or mutilation

6. Children will present with a particular injury pattern and physiologic response to trauma. These responses may vary depending upon the child's: (C 6-1.2)

    a. size
    b. level of maturation
    c. overall development
    d. all of the above

7. The EMT should frequently reassess the injured infant or child since they can compensate for a serious injury longer than an adult. (C 6-1.3)

    a. true
    b. false

8. A foreign body airway obstruction should be suspected if an infant or child suddenly develops respiratory distress with coughing, gagging, stridor (high-pitched sound caused by an obstruction in the trachea), or wheezing. (C 6-1.6)

    a. true
    b. false

9. Management strategies specific to respiratory distress or failure include all of the following **except:** (C 6-1.7)

    a. Maintain proficiency in infant and child CPR and techniques for clearing an obstructed airway.
    b. Always examine the throat of a child who is complaining with sore throat and/or difficulty swallowing
    c. Select airway and respiratory adjuncts based on the size of the patient and the ventilatory support needed.
    d. Only use a BVM that delivers at least 450 cc of air to provide the full-term infant or child with an adequate tidal volume.

10. Remember to have suction equipment available as pediatric patients are prone to vomiting. (C 6-1.7)

    a. true
    b. false

11. Signs of shock include which of the following: (C 6-1.8)

    a. altered level of consciousness
    b. increased respiratory rate, rapid heart rate
    c. cool or cold clammy skin, prolonged capillary refill
    d. all of the above

12. Inadequate organ tissue perfusion is indicated by all of the following signs **except:** (C 6-1.9)

    a. a change in the level of consciousness
    b. increased heart rate
    c. a normal blood pressure
    d. increased capillary refill time

13. Most pediatric patients go into cardiac arrest as a result of ventricular fibrillation, therefore defibrillation is a primary skill in pediatric resuscitation. (C 6-1.10)

    a. true
    b. false

14. Causes of seizures include all of the following **except:** (C 6-1.11)

    a. abnormal electrical activity in the brain
    b. elevated body temperature (fever)
    c. hypoxia, head trauma
    d. high blood sugar levels

15. _____ is the period immediately preceding the seizure wherein the patient experiences a certain feeling or sensation that warns of an impending seizure. (C 6-1.12)

    a. Postictal
    b. Preictal
    c. Aura
    d. Lethargy

16. In treating a seizure victim, the EMT should use all of the following management techniques **except:** (C 6-1.12)

    a. the child should be gently assisted to a side-lying position with special consideration given to airway patency
    b. the area should be cleared of hazardous items that might cause injury during the seizure activity
    c. insert a wooden spoon into the mouth if the teeth are clenched
    d. a nasal airway is an appropriate alternative adjunct for this situation

17. Injury patterns in children and adult patients differ due to which of the following factors: (C 6-1.13)

    a. the child is smaller than an adult and is therefore prone to a wider range of injuries
    b. in infants and younger children, the head is larger in proportion to the rest of the body
    c. the child's skeleton is not completely calcified and has many active growth centers
    d. all of the above

18. The primary treatment goal for the infant and child trauma patient in the field is: (C 6-1.14)

    a. rapid transport to definitive care at the hospital
    b. to decrease scene time to 1/2 of the time spent with the adult patient
    c. to provide high-concentration oxygen after transport is initiated
    d. rapid transport to an appropriate facility as a secondary concern with the infant or child patient

19. Status epilepticus is a continuous seizure or a series of seizures in which the patient does not regain consciousness. (C 6-1.12)

    a. true
    b. false

20. Indicators of child abuse include: (C 6-1.15)

    a. bruises or burns in patterns that suggest intentional infliction
    b. injuries in various stages of healing
    c. children under 2 years of age with multiple fractures
    d. all of the above

21. When reporting suspected child abuse, as may be required by state law, the EMT should report: (C 6-1.16)

    a. what he or she sees
    b. what he or she hears
    c. what he or she thinks
    d. a and b

22. In dealing with suspected child abuse situations, important roles for the EMT-B include: (C 6-1.16)

    a. be nonjudgmental
    b. do not accuse anyone of child abuse even though it may appear obvious to you
    c. carefully document in objective terms exactly what you see or have assessed on the child
    d. all of the above

23. The EMT should consider participating in a debriefing session after dealing with a critical infant or child transport. (C 6-1.17)

    a. true
    b. false

24. Providing emotional support to the pediatric patient and the family can make an emergency scenario more tolerable for everyone. (A 6-1.19)

    a. true
    b. false

25. The first sign of respiratory distress in an infant is usually: (C 6-1.5)

    a. a rapid rate of breathing
    b. a decreased pulse rate
    c. a decreased capillary refill time
    d. increased thirst

Scenario

Read each scenario. Write the answers to the corresponding questions in the space provided.

SCENARIO #1:

It is a quiet Sunday afternoon in the early fall. You and your partner are preparing for the continuing education class that is scheduled to be taught at the station tomorrow night.

Suddenly the phone rings and the dispatcher directs you to the scene where a child is bleeding. According to the parents, the 9-month-old child fell off of the kitchen cabinet while trying to get to the cookie jar.

Upon arrival at the scene, you immediately note old bruises on the patient's trunk, and abrasions in various stages of healing. There are two small lacerations on each thigh that are bleeding moderately and a large scalp laceration that is bleeding profusely.

continued

1. How would you assess this patient?

_____

_____

_____

_____

2. What interventions would you perform?

_____

_____

_____

_____

3. List three transport considerations.

_____

_____

_____

_____

4. State at least two considerations when documenting and reporting this incident.

_____

_____

_____

_____

CHAPTER 35 ANSWERS TO REVIEW QUESTIONS

1. c	6. d	11. d	16. c	21. d
2. d	7. a	12. c	17. d	22. d
3. c	8. a	13. b	18. a	23. a
4. b	9. b	14. d	19. a	24. a
5. c	10. a	15. c	20. d	25. a

SCENARIO SOLUTIONS

Scenario #1:

1. Assessment of this patient should progress as follows:

- Perform an initial assessment and physical exam in an area away from the parents, if possible.
- Assess level of consciousness, maintain C-spine control
- Assess airway, breathing, circulation
- Complete spinal packaging

2. The interventions to be performed are as follows:
   - Control bleeding
   - Administer oxygen
   - Gather pertinent past medical history

3. The following are transport considerations:
   - Treat this case as a "load and go."
   - Monitor the child's airway and observe for further signs of abuse en route to the hospital.
   - Cleanse the lacerations and place a bandage on the thigh injuries.

4. To document and report this incident:
   - Report and discuss this case with the proper authorities
   - Document and report only what you see or hear
   - Remain nonjudgemental
   - Document facts, not opinions

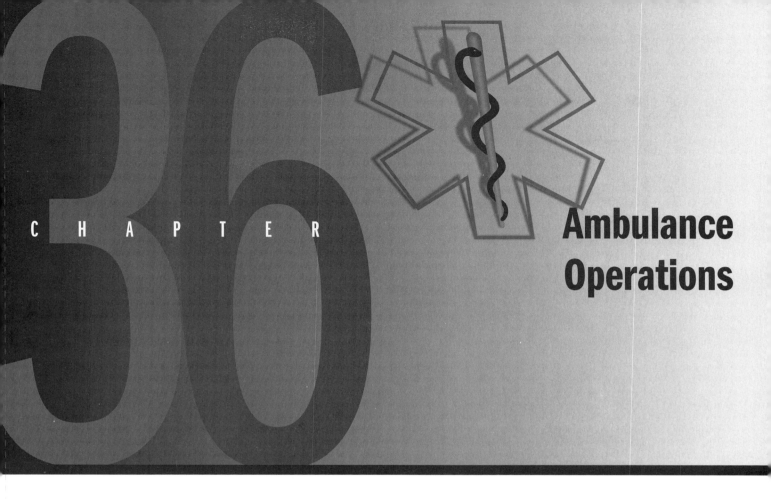

CHAPTER 36

Ambulance Operations

Reading Assignment: Chapter 36, pgs. 683–704

OBJECTIVES

1. Identify the medical and nonmedical equipment needed to respond to a call.

2. List the phases of an ambulance call.

3. Describe the general provisions of state laws relating to the operation of an emergency vehicle, including:
   - speed
   - warning lights
   - right-of-way
   - parking
   - turning

4. List contributing factors to unsafe driving conditions.

5. Describe the considerations that should be given to:
   - requests for escorts
   - following an escort vehicle
   - intersections

6. Describe the concept of "due regard for safety of others" while operating an emergency vehicle.

7. Identify the essential information for responding to a call.

8. Identify factors that may affect response to a call.

9. Summarize the importance of preparing the unit for the next response.

10. Distinguish between the terms *cleaning*, *disinfection*, *high-level disinfection*, and *sterilization* and the application of these following patient care.

11. Explain the rationale for having the unit prepared to respond.

INTRODUCTION

Knowledge of ambulance operations is applied throughout the career of the EMT-B. The ambulance is one of the vital links in the chain of resources necessary to deliver emergency medical care in the prehospital environment.

Although some EMT-Bs may never actually work on a transporting unit, they must be prepared to respond and render care under a variety of situations. The ambulance and the associated equipment must be maintained in safe, working condition. The EMT who attempts to render care with malfunctioning equipment may harm the patient.

Operators of the ambulance must have knowledge of the local laws governing the safe operation of an ambulance. Knowledge of these laws enables the driver to operate the ambulance safely and accomplish the mission of EMS.

REVIEW QUESTIONS

Please circle one correct answer for each question.

1. The largest and most complex piece of EMS equipment is the: (C 7-1.1)

   a. cot
   b. defibrillator
   c. ambulance
   d. mobile radio

2. An ambulance is designed to get EMTs and equipment to the emergency scene safely and to transport patients to a medical facility. (C 7-1.1)

   a. true
   b. false

3. The Type I ambulance has: (C 7-1.1)

   a. a conventional cab
   b. a chassis with a modular ambulance body
   c. no passageway between the patient's and driver's compartment, other than a window
   d. all of the above

4. The Type II ambulance is essentially a converted van, usually with a raised roof. The driver and patient area form an integral unit. (C 7-1.1)

   a. true
   b. false

5. Commonly, the Type III ambulance is mounted on a van chassis and a walkway or passage connects the patient compartment and the driver's compartment. The Type III ambulance is similar to: (C 7-1.1)

   a. the Type I
   b. the Type II
   c. both Type I and II
   d. none of the above

6. The General Services Administration has established specifications for ambulances purchased by the Federal Government. These standards have been adopted by many state and local jurisdictions and are known as the: (C 7-1.1 and 7-1.3)

   a. ABC standards
   b. ICC standards
   c. KKK standards
   d. AAA standards

7. Factors that may dictate different quantities and kinds of equipment carried in the ambulance include all of the following **except:** (C 7-1.1)

   a. the type of service normally delivered in your area
   b. the transport times
   c. local statutes or regulations
   d. the average age of clients

8. All of the following supplies are considered basic supplies **except:** (C 7-1.1)

   a. pillows (disposable or nondisposable)
   b. blankets (disposable or nondisposable)
   c. defibrillator
   d. emesis bags/basins (disposable)

9. Biohazard disposal bags are an example of equipment that is: (C 7-1.13)

   a. FCC compliant
   b. OSHA compliant
   c. FDA compliant
   d. NIH compliant

10. All of the following are examples of items necessary to monitor a patient's condition **except:** (C 7-1.1)

    a. sphygmomanometers (blood pressure cuff)
    b. stethoscopes
    c. flow meters
    d. thermometers (disposable)

11. Nonmedical equipment includes: (C 7-1.1)

    a. safety equipment
    b. equipment used to extricate victims
    c. preplanned routes and comprehensive street maps
    d. all of the above

12. A variety of emergency vehicle driving courses are offered. These courses have been developed by all of the following **except:** (C 7-1.6)

    a. Department of Transportation (DOT)
    b. The National Safety Council
    c. insurance companies
    d. National Ambulance Alliance

13. Duties of the EMT when preparing to respond to emergency calls include all of the following **except:** (C 7-1.11)

    a. assuring that his partner has prepared the ambulance
    b. assuring that the unit is in safe operating condition
    c. assuring that the necessary equipment is available
    d. identify repairs and maintenance needed

14. Daily vehicle inspection is considered to be part of an ambulance call. (C 7-1.2)

    a. true
    b. false

15. The dispatch center serves all of the following functions **except:** (C 7-1.7)

    a. provides a connection between the public and the EMS system
    b. receives calls for assistance
    c. dispatches the necessary personnel
    d. always provides initial, verbal, emergency care instructions over the phone

16. Seat belts are needed for all occupants of the emergency vehicle. (C 7-1.3)

    a. true
    b. false

17. Factors that can contribute to unsafe driving conditions include all of the following **except:** (C 7-1.4)

    a. ice
    b. hurricanes
    c. the time of day or day of the week
    d. preplanned route

18. Factors that may affect response to a call include: (C 7-1.4)

    a. an uncooperative motorist
    b. day of the week
    c. time of day
    d. all of the above

19. It is the driver's responsibility to operate the ambulance with due regard for the safety of others. (C 7-1.6)

    a. true
    b. false

20. Use of lights and sirens does not in any way exempt an emergency vehicle operator from the requirement to drive with due regard for the safety of others. (C 7-1.3 and C 7-1.6)

    a. true
    b. false

21. Should escorts be needed, the ability to communicate with the escorting units will increase the safety of the escort. (C 7-1.5)

    a. true
    b. false

22. In cases of unstable trauma, rapid transport to the receiving facility is the most beneficial treatment. Splinting of major fractures should be done: (C 7-1.9)

    a. while transport is being undertaken
    b. before transport
    c. at the hospital
    d. by the senior EMT at the scene

23. A PCR should include: (C 7-1.10)

    a. mechanism of injury, illness, or both
    b. injuries found and treatments
    c. vital signs
    d. all of the above

24. Essentials for completing a call upon arrival at the emergency department include all of the following **except:** (C 7-1.12)

    a. make a verbal report to the medical staff
    b. follow up with a written report of the call
    c. transfer the patient's effects to the medical staff
    d. submit a copy of the PCR to law enforcement officers

25. When cleaning the ambulance, particularly the patient compartment, it is essential that the EMT dispose of any biohazards properly. (C 7-1.14)

    a. true
    b. false

Scenario

Read each scenario. Write the answers to the corresponding questions in the space provided.

SCENARIO #1:

You and your partner are beginning your duty day. As they were leaving, the previous crew told you that one of the units had a near empty tank because they had been too busy to refuel.

You and your partner complete the checks of the trucks and find that the low fuel in one unit is the only problem area. You elect to fill the tank when you go out to lunch.

One hour after your duty shift begins, you are dispatched to the scene of a multi-victim MVA that requires that all your units respond. The location of the accident is 15 miles away from the station and 20 miles away from the nearest receiving medical facility. You realize immediately that the unit with the near empty tank cannot be used in this call.

continued

1. What should you have done to prepare for your shift prior to this first call?

_____

_____

_____

_____

2. What are your and your partner's responsibilities regarding vehicle check and maintenance?

_____

_____

_____

_____

CHAPTER 36 ANSWERS TO REVIEW QUESTIONS

1.	c	6.	c	11.	d	16.	a	21.	a
2.	a	7.	d	12.	d	17.	d	22.	a
3.	d	8.	c	13.	a	18.	d	23.	d
4.	a	9.	b	14.	a	19.	a	24.	d
5.	a	10.	c	15.	d	20.	a	25.	a

SCENARIO SOLUTIONS

Scenario #1:

1. You should have arranged to put fuel in the ambulance immediately following your daily inspection.

2. You and your partner both have the duty to check out the ambulance and equipment immediately after reporting to work. While conducting the routine daily inspection, you and your partner go over the equipment and make corrections and adjustments as indicated.

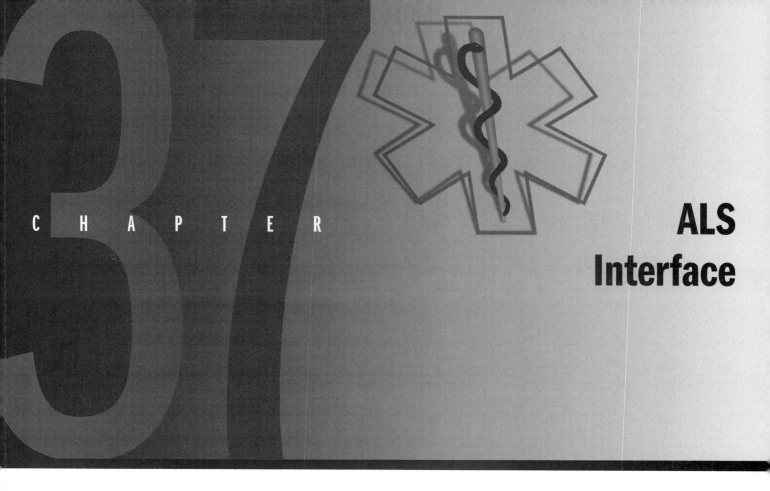

CHAPTER 37

ALS Interface

Reading Assignment: Chapter 37, pgs. 705–714

OBJECTIVES

1. Define the need for ALS interface.

2. Demonstrate the decision-making process for using ALS interface.

3. Identify the circumstances under which ALS interface is appropriate.

4. Define the need for good communication and interpersonal skills.

INTRODUCTION

This chapter examines the decision-making process, from the perspective of the EMT-B provider, regarding interface with advanced providers of prehospital care. This interface is often necessary to provide advanced levels of prehospital care for some patients. Emergency medical technicians use acquired skills and knowledge to decide when the need for advanced levels of care are appropriate in the prehospital setting.

REVIEW QUESTIONS

Please circle one correct answer for each question.

1. Prehospital ALS functions as an extension of a: (Chp. Obj. #2)
   a. licensed physician
   b. state governing body
   c. registered nurse
   d. paramedic

2. Invasive procedures, whether performed under indirect medical control or direct medical control, are ultimately accountable to the: (Chp. Obj. #2)
   a. trauma nurse
   b. nurse practitioner
   c. lead paramedic
   d. medical control physician

3. Prehospital ALS does not act as an independent authority to provide invasive procedures that constitute ALS. (Chp. Obj. #2)
   a. true
   b. false

4. Written guidelines delineating procedures that may be performed without direct physician contact are called: (Chp. Obj. #2)
   a. protocols
   b. standing orders
   c. guidelines
   d. procedures

5. The structure that allows the prehospital ALS providers to act on behalf of the physician is termed: (Chp. Obj. #2)
   a. standard practice
   b. medical control
   c. judicial control
   d. executive control

6. To assist in determining the need for ALS assistance, the EMT should consider all of the following conditions as possible criteria **except:** (Chp. Obj. #1)
   a. patient condition warrants a level of care beyond your capability
   b. multiple trauma involving extrication greater than 10 minutes
   c. chest pain with signs, symptoms, or both indicative of myocardial infarction (MI) or heart attack
   d. respiratory rate of 12-24 breaths/min

7. Once the need for ALS interface is determined, the request must be made: (Chp. Obj. #1)
   a. within the first hour
   b. after transport is initiated
   c. as soon as possible
   d. prior to dispatch

8. Consideration for ALS interface must include: (Chp. Obj. #3)

   a. preparation for transport
   b. selecting an appropriate intercept site
   c. availability of ALS units
   d. all of the above

9. Situations warranting the use of ALS include: (Chp. Obj. #3)

   a. heart attack
   b. cardiac arrest
   c. respiratory arrest
   d. all of the above

10. The overall purpose of ALS is to afford patients advanced levels of care appropriate to their condition in a timely manner. (Chp. Obj. #3)

    a. true
    b. false

11. An important consideration in determining the risk-benefit of ALS rather than direct transport to the hospital is: (Chp. Obj. #3)

    a. time
    b. availability
    c. environmental conditions
    d. all of the above

12. Advanced life support should be requested if the need exists for ALS intervention and the time of arrival or intercept is shorter than the time required for direct transport to the hospital. (Chp. Obj. #3)

    a. true
    b. false

13. The key to effective interagency, multi-level patient care is: (Chp. Obj. #4)

    a. communication
    b. education
    c. legislation
    d. logistics

14. Information garnered by the EMT regarding the patient must be communicated to the ALS provider. These information items include: (Chp. Obj. #4)

    a. patient history
    b. vital signs
    c. present illness or injury
    d. all of the above

15. It is the responsibility of the EMT to follow an established patient presentation to facilitate followup care by both the ALS provider and the EMT. (Chp. Obj. #2)

    a. true
    b. false

16. Useful concepts in communication skills include all of the following **except:** (Chp. Obj. #2)

    a. present patient information clearly and concisely
    b. be prepared to repeat specific details
    c. use discretion when nonEMS personnel are present
    d. disregarding patient history

17. The EMT must remember that family members deserve consideration and should use discretion when discussing the patient's condition in their presence. (Chp. Obj. #4)

    a. true
    b. false

18. There may be times when conflict arises between the EMT and ALS providers at the scene of a prehospital emergency. The person who assumes medical supervision and responsibility for the patient is the: (Chp. Obj. #4)

    a. EMT-B
    b. first responder
    c. ALS provider
    d. law enforcement officer

19. Conflicts between EMTs and ALS providers should be resolved in a calm, professional manner outside of the scene. (Chp. Obj. #4)

    a. true
    b. false

20. EMTs must realize that calling for ALS intervention is a positive action and exemplifies their understanding of the prime objective of quality patient care. (Chp. Obj. #4)

    a. true
    b. false

Scenario

Read each scenario. Write the answers to the corresponding questions in the space provided.

SCENARIO #1:

You and your EMT crew are dispatched to a call for a person who is "feeling sick." Upon arrival you find a 36-year-old male who informs you that he was stung by a wasp. He is complaining of a tight feeling in his chest and is experiencing difficulty breathing. Secondary complaints include nausea, vomiting, dizziness, and feeling "hot all over."

Dispatch informs you that an ALS unit is within three blocks of your location and is available at your request. You realize that transport time to the hospital from your location is approximately 10 minutes.

1. Does the patient's condition meet the suggested criteria for ALS?

_____

_____

_____

_____

continued

2. Is ALS available in a shorter period of time than transport time to the hospital?

_____

_____

_____

_____

3. Who assumes care for the patient when the ALS provider arrives?

_____

_____

_____

4. While awaiting the arrival of ALS providers, what should the EMT-B accomplish?

_____

_____

_____

_____

CHAPTER 37 ANSWERS TO REVIEW QUESTIONS

1. a	4. b	8. d	12. a	16. d	20. a
2. d	3. a	7. c	11. d	15. a	19. a
	6. d	10. a	14. d	18. c
5. b	9. d	13. a	17. a

SCENARIO SOLUTIONS

Scenario #1

1. Yes. The patient is presenting with signs and symptoms indicative of a severe allergic reaction. It is also clear that this patient will benefit from ALS interventions in addition to those instituted by the EMT.
2. Yes. The patient will receive ALS interventions in 2–4 minutes from the ALS providers compared to the 10 minutes required to get the patient to the hospital for ALS.
3. The ALS provider will assume care for the patient upon arrival at the scene.
4. Initial appropriate interventions and preparation for transport should begin.

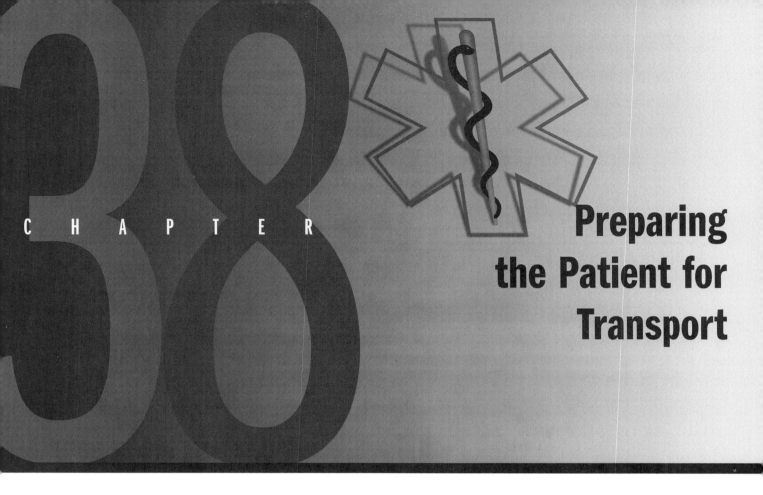

CHAPTER 38

Preparing the Patient for Transport

Reading Assigment: Chapter 38, pgs. 715–726

OBJECTIVES

1. Describe time-dependent medical problems as they relate to trauma patients and medical patients.

2. Discuss risk-benefit ratios in prehospital care as they relate to trauma patients and medical patients.

3. Explain why transport is often the most important intervention in prehospital care.

4. List the different phases of patient assessment.

5. List the factors to be considered when assessing the trauma patient for prompt transport.

INTRODUCTION

This chapter focuses on many of the issues that should be considered to transport emergency patients promptly and safely. The EMT should understand the general principles regarding preparation for transport.

Definitive care of emergency patients takes place within the confines of the hospital. Prompt transport remains one of the most important therapeutic interventions in emergency care. The goal in most patient encounters is efficient evaluation, stabilization, and packaging of the patient for transport. The decision making involved in preparing for transport can sometimes be one of the most complex issues facing prehospital providers.

A variety of factors that often are not under the control of EMTs influence transport decisions. Such factors may include access to the patient, scene safety, availability of personnel or other resources, type of medical problem, and others. Every effort should be made to minimize prehospital time without adversely affecting the patient.

REVIEW QUESTIONS

Please circle one correct answer for each question.

1. The effectiveness of many medical interventions is related to the time at which they are implemented. (Chp. Obj. #1)
   a. true
   b. false

2. One of the most important interventions in prehospital care is transport; the benefits of all other interventions must be weighed against the risks of delaying transport. (Chp. Obj. #3)
   a. true
   b. false

3. In the prehospital setting, information regarding the patient complaint begins flowing into the system at the time of: (Chp. Obj. #5)
   a. notification of medical control
   b. occurrence of the incident
   c. dispatch
   d. transport

4. The earliest point at which the EMTs can begin assessing patient needs is: (Chp. Obj. #4)
   a. during dispatch
   b. upon arrival at the scene
   c. while en route to the scene
   d. during transport

5. Prearrival assessment and planning involve a discussion between responding EMTs regarding the: (Chp. Obj. #4)
   a. role of each responder
   b. anticipated equipment needs
   c. scene management
   d. all of the above

6. Factors that must be considered when evaluating and packaging the trauma patient for transport include all of the following **except:** (Chp. Obj. #5)
   a. mechanism of injury
   b. severity of injury
   c. delayed life threats
   d. transport time

7. Treatment of medical conditions can last from minutes to hours, to days or weeks. (Chp. Obj. #1)

   a. true
   b. false

8. A patient who presents in cardiac arrest from acute myocardial infarction (AMI) must be assessed and treated: (Chp. Obj. #1)

   a. two hours from onset of symptoms
   b. promptly upon arrival at the scene
   c. after arrival at the hospital
   d. only during transport

9. If the initial assessment of a patient raises suspicion of a life-threatening injury such as uncontrolled bleeding, scene times should be maximized. (Chp. Obj. #5)

   a. true
   b. false

10. Virtually every treatment or intervention that is administered to a patient has an associated risk-benefit ratio. (Chp. Obj. #2)

    a. true
    b. false

11. Reliance on input from local medical control is useful in defining which interventions should be done on and off the scene. (Chp. Obj. #2)

    a. true
    b. false

12. The initial dispatch information relayed to the responding EMS unit is a vital part of the: (Chp. Obj. #4)

    a. definitive care
    b. predispatch
    c. patient assessment
    d. postdispatch

13. With the advent of prearrival instructions being given by dispatchers, patient assessment and even treatment can now be started directly from the dispatch center. (Chp. Obj. #4)

    a. true
    b. false

14. Information gathered at the scene may be provided to the EMT by: (Chp. Obj. #5)

    a. police officers
    b. family members
    c. the patient
    d. all of the above

15. In dealing with the trauma patient, factors that will influence the amount of time and stabilization required on the scene include: (Chp. Obj. #5)

    a. mechanism of injury, barriers at the scene
    b. severity of injury, training level of other providers
    c. immediate life threats, transport time
    d. all of the above

16. Immediate life threats in onscene trauma management are primarily: (Chp. Obj. #5)

   a. airway problems
   b. external arterial bleeding
   c. alteration in level of consciousness
   d. all of the above

17. A good working knowledge of the capabilities of the local EMS system will dictate whether the patient is transported directly to a hospital or an ALS intercept is made. (Chp. Obj. #3)

   a. true
   b. false

18. Most poisonings are time dependent and if the patient is unstable, transport should be initiated immediately just as if the patient were a trauma patient losing blood. (Chp. Obj. #3)

   a. true
   b. false

19. Risk-benefit ratio in prehospital care refers to weighing the risk of delaying transport against the benefit of performing the intervention on the scene. (Chp. Obj. #2)

   a. true
   b. false

20. The ultimate goal in managing the trauma patient is to: (Chp. Obj. #5)

   a. render definitive care in the field
   b. move the patient to a definitive care facility
   c. efficiently coordinate the bystanders on the scene
   d. perform all assessment en route

Scenario

Read each scenario. Write the answers to the corresponding questions in the space provided.

SCENARIO #1:

Fortunately, all is quiet on this cold, rainy night. You have been studying for the upcoming hazardous material (HAZMAT) course at your local station. Suddenly, you and your EMT-B partner are called to respond to the scene of a motorcycle crash.

The location of the crash is in a rural area, approximately 12 miles outside of town. Law officers are on the scene. Your dispatch information en route indicates that there are two victims involved. One victim is unconscious. The other victim is alert and walking about the scene.

1. What transport decisions can be made at the time of dispatch?

   _____

   _____

   _____

   _____

continued

2. En route to the scene, what further decisions can be made?

_____

_____

_____

_____

CHAPTER 38 ANSWERS TO REVIEW QUESTIONS

1. a	5. d	9. b	13. a	17. a
2. a	6. c	10. a	14. d	18. a
3. c	7. a	11. a	15. d	19. a
4. a	8. b	12. c	16. d	20. b

SCENARIO SOLUTIONS

Scenario #1

1. Based on weather conditions and interstate location, any patients found will be rapidly prepared for transport.

2. Based on the information received en route to the accident, several issues should be considered before arrival on the scene. There are two patients and at least one additional ambulance may be required for transport. Consider that ALS providers may be needed at the scene. Given the location of the crash, helicopter transport should be considered if available. More personnel may be needed since both patients may be critically injured.

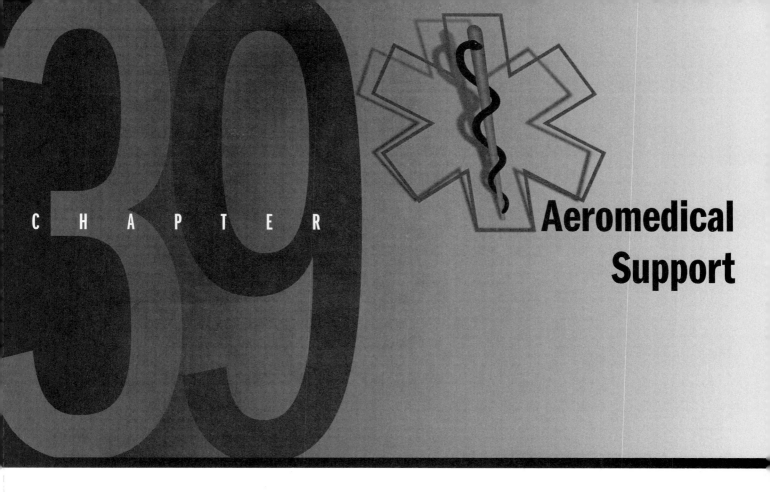

CHAPTER 39

Aeromedical Support

Reading Assignment: Chapter 39, pgs. 727–740

OBJECTIVES

1. Describe the factors that may indicate the need for aeromedical transportation.

2. Identify the steps necessary to prepare a safe landing zone.

3. Identify the steps to guide a helicopter to the landing zone.

4. Demonstrate how to operate near an aircraft safely.

5. List the steps taken to prepare a patient for air transport.

INTRODUCTION

This chapter discusses the use of aeromedical transport. It also describes how aeromedical transport can greatly affect the survival of the patient. Key issues discussed in this chapter include the importance of knowing when to request aeromedical transport, how to work safely around an aircraft and proper preparation of the patient for the flight.

REVIEW QUESTIONS

Please circle one correct answer for each question.

1. Helicopter rotor blades can range from 3 to 15 ft off the ground. (Chp. Obj. #2)

   (a) true
   b. false

2. Which of the following guidelines can be used to evaluate the need for aeromedical services? (Chp. Obj. #1)

   a. mechanism of injury
   b. the physical findings
   c. special situations
   (d) all of the above

3. Which of the following mechanisms of injury may not indicate the need for aeromedical transportation? (Chp. Obj. #1)

   (a) a person falls 5 ft
   b. a person is ejected from a vehicle
   c. a pedestrian is struck by a motor vehicle
   d. a person in an MVA with speeds greater than 25 mph

4. Which of the following physical exam findings does not indicate the need for aeromedical transportation? (Chp. Obj. #1)

   a. a head injury with a decrease in the LOC
   b. a penetrating wound to the chest or abdomen
   c. an airway that needs advanced procedures to be maintained
   (d) isolated fracture of the radius and ulna, pulses present

5. Which of the following circumstances and patient medical conditions may warrant the use of aeromedical support? (Chp. Obj. #1)

   a. certain obstetrical emergencies with a long ground transport time
   b. unexpected or complicated premature deliveries with a long ground transport time
   c. medical problems that require ALS and none is available by ground
   (d) all of the above

6. What are the two phases of activating aeromedical support? (Chp. Obj. #2)

   a. standby and transport
   (b) standby and response
   c. standdown and response
   d. response and transport

7. When should an aeromedical team be asked to respond to a scene? (Chp. Obj. #1)

   a. when the initial call is received from bystanders
   (b) when the situation has been identified by on-scene personnel and meets the criteria for aeromedical support
   c. when first responders state that it sounds like a bad call
   d. when the patient requests air transport

8. Early recognition and activation of aeromedical transport are essential in critically ill and injured patients, and decreasing the amount of time before hospital arrival can save a life. (Chp. Obj. #1)

   a. true
   b. false

9. What are the minimum landing zone dimensions for helicopters during daylight hours? (Chp. Obj. #2)

   a. 60 ft × 60 ft
   b. 30 ft × 60 ft
   c. 40 ft × 60 ft
   d. 100 ft × 100 ft

10. What are the minimum landing zone dimensions for helicopters during nighttime operations? (Chp. Obj. #2)

   a. 60 ft × 60 ft
   b. 30 ft × 60 ft
   c. 40 ft × 60 ft
   d. 100 ft × 100 ft

11. Which of the following are landing zone hazards? (Chp. Obj. #2)

   a. wires
   b. debris
   c. unmarked towers or poles
   d. all of the above

12. When a landing zone is marked with flares, a flare should be placed in the middle of the zone as a reference point for the pilot. (Chp. Obj. #3)

   a. true
   b. false

13. Bright lights pointed at the landing zone will help the pilot's night vision. (Chp. Obj. #3)

   a. true
   b. false

14. When giving landing instructions to the helicopter pilot, always use references in relationship to the aircraft. (Chp. Obj. #4)

   a. true
   b. false

15. Which of the following is a safety violation when working around a helicopter? (Chp. Obj. #4)

   a. approaching the helicopter from the rear
   b. approaching the helicopter from the front
   c. parking a vehicle 100 ft from the aircraft
   d. approaching from the downhill side of the aircraft

16. The loading or unloading of a helicopter with the rotor system turning is called a "hot load" and is considered a very safe procedure. (Chp. Obj. #4)

   a. true
   b. false

17. Which of the following patient care interventions should be performed before loading a patient into the helicopter? (Chp. Obj. #5)

    a. ensure adequate airway control, breathing and circulation
    b. treat life-threatening injuries
    c. place the patient on oxygen
    d. all of the above

18. When considering the physiology of gases, which of the following are true? (Chp. Obj. #5)

    a. at higher altitudes gases compress and concentrations of oxygen decrease
    b. at higher altitudes gases expand and concentrations of oxygen increase
    c. at higher altitudes gases expand and concentrations of oxygen decrease
    d. at higher altitudes gases compress and concentrations of oxygen increase

19. Which of the following might be considered advantages of air transportation as compared to ground transportation? (Chp. Obj. #1)

    a. rapid transportation
    b. transportation not affected by roads, traffic, or terrain
    c. air transport staffed with advanced personnel and equipment that is often not available on ground units
    d. all of the above

20. Which of the following is not a function of the standby phase? (Chp. Obj. #1)

    a. preparation of the aircraft
    b. transport of the aeromedical team to the scene
    c. locating the incident by the communications specialist
    d. checking the weather conditions by the pilot

Scenario

Read each scenario. Write the answers to the corresponding questions in the space provided.

SCENARIO #1:

The Saturday evening local college football game ended 30 minutes ago and traffic is horrendous! You and your partner receive a call to an MVA involving five vehicles on an interstate approximately 10 miles from the stadium.

Based on the initial reports from law enforcement officers, there are multiple injuries and all lanes of traffic are blocked. The local trauma center is 5 miles away by ground. Your dispatcher notifies you that a helicopter has been placed on standby.

continued

1. How should you determine the patient transport mode and the necessity for aeromedical response?

    _____

    _____

    _____

2. What types of backup units will you consider summoning to the scene?

    _____

    _____

    _____

3. List at least five considerations regarding the landing zone to be established.

    _____

    _____

    _____

    _____

4. List at least four considerations regarding preparation of patients for aeromedical transport.

    _____

    _____

    _____

    _____

CHAPTER 39 ANSWERS TO REVIEW QUESTIONS

1. a	5. d	9. a	13. b	17. d
2. d	6. b	10. d	14. a	18. c
3. a	7. b	11. d	15. a	19. d
4. d	8. a	12. b	16. b	20. b

SCENARIO SOLUTIONS

Scenario #1

1. From the initial reports of the incident, you and your partner realize the seriousness and potential hazards of the incident. The determination regarding patient transport mode (ground transport vs. aeromedical transport) is based upon:

    • the number of victims
    • the seriousness of the injuries
    • access time to definitive care

2. Consider summoning the following backup units:

- rescue-extrication teams
- ALS units
- fire department units
- BLS units
- number of aeromedical teams
- multiple-casualty incident (MCI) manager

3. The following landing zone considerations need to be established:

- proximity to incident site
- hazards near the scene
- weather conditions
- need for flat area, 100×100 ft.
- area free from obstacles (i.e. electrical wires, trees, etc.)

4. To prepare the patient for aeromedical transport:

- initiate patient care by ground crew
- ensure adequate airway control, breathing, and circulation
- treat life-threatening injuries
- initiate oxygen therapy
- immobilize spine per local protocol
- transfer patient to air crew properly

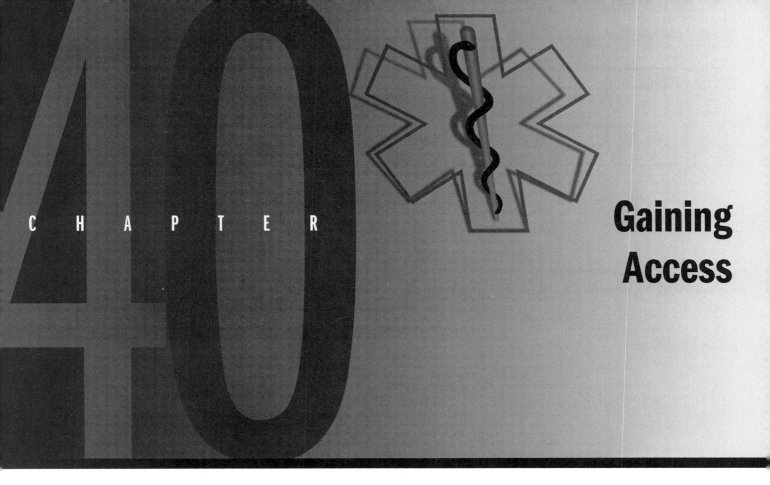

CHAPTER 40

Gaining Access

Reading Assignment: Chapter 40, pgs. 741–752

OBJECTIVES

1. Describe the types of rescue operations.
2. Describe the types of rescue vehicles.
3. Describe the priorities of rescue.
4. Describe the purpose of extrication.
5. Explain how the EMT prepares for the run.
6. Describe preplanning and size-up.
7. Discuss the role of the EMT in extrication.
8. Describe the safety procedures for the EMT and the victim including personal safety equipment.
9. Define the fundamental components of extrication.
10. Describe and evaluate various methods of gaining access from simple to complex.
11. Describe the actions necessary after the rescue operation concludes.

▮ INTRODUCTION

Emergency medical technicians often respond to incidents where one or more patients are trapped. The EMT's primary responsibility, after ensuring his or her own safety, is assessment and stabilization of the patient. Gaining access to the patient often requires imagination and ingenuity.

This chapter discusses elements of a successful rescue operation, as well as planning and training. It also describes scene size-up, safety, and the fundamental components of extrication.

▮ REVIEW QUESTIONS

Please circle one correct answer for each question.

1. The most common type of entrapment occurs as a result of automobile collisions. (C 7-2.4)
   a. true
   b. false

2. At the scene of a MVA, the EMT's responsibility is the patient, not the extrication. (C 7-2.2)
   a. true
   b. false

3. An ambulance that carries simple extrication tools would be classified as a: (C 7-2.7)
   a. light duty rescue unit
   b. extrication truck
   c. medium duty rescue unit
   d. specialized unit

4. Disentanglement involves removal of the wreckage from around the victim so that emergency care can be provided. (C 7-2.4)
   a. true
   b. false

5. _____ involves actual removal of the patient from the vehicle. (C 7-2.4)
   a. Disentanglement
   b. Entrapment
   c. Extrication
   d. Excavation

6. The EMT's primary responsibility at an incident where one or more victims is trapped is: (C 7-2.2)
   a. rapid and safe disentanglement and extrication
   b. providing emergency care while specially trained personnel perform extrication
   c. traffic control
   d. triage

7. Water rescue is a type of rescue operation that involves a patient who is trapped in water or in a position in which he or she cannot be reached without crossing a significant body of water. (C 7-2.4)

    ⓐ true
    b. false

8. Water rescue simply requires the ability of the rescuer to swim and should, therefore, be attempted routinely by EMTs. (C 7-2.3)

    a. true
    ⓑ false

9. High-angle rescue is a type of rescue that involves a victim who is in a position or place far off the ground. Examples of high-angle rescue include: (C 7-2.3)

    a. a high-rise building under construction
    b. a ski lift or a water tower
    c. the ledge of a sheer rock wall
    ⓓ all of the above

10. A cave-in occurs when rock or earth collapses around and traps a victim. It can occur in: (C 7-2.4)

    a. caves
    b. construction sites
    c. utility trenches
    ⓓ all of the above

11. Complex vehicle rescue requires specialized equipment. All of the following are examples of this type of equipment **except:** (C 7-2.7)

    a. port-a-powers
    b. powered hydraulic spreaders and cutters
    ⓒ hammer
    d. hydraulic rams

12. Dive equipment and rigging/rapelling equipment are two types of equipment found on heavy rescue units. (C 7-2.6)

    ⓐ true
    b. false

13. Moderately pinned victims may need specialized tools to remove them, but the extrication can usually be accomplished in a minimum amount of time. (C 7-2.4)

    ⓐ true
    b. false

14. During any extrication operations, the primary functions of the EMT are to: (C 7-2.2)

    a. locate victims
    b. triage
    c. treat the victims of the accident
    ⓓ all of the above

15. Which of the following is not considered appropriate protective equipment for EMT safety? (C 7-2.3)

    a. turnout gear
    b. a heavy, fire-resistant coat
    c. tennis shoes
    d. helmet

16. When considering which window to break to gain access to the patient, the EMT should do all of the following **except:** (C 7-2.5)

    a. determine which window is the furthest from the victim
    b. determine which window is large enough to accommodate safe entry of the EMT
    c. cover the patient with a blanket to prevent injury
    d. always gain access through the back windshield

17. Always try the simple approach to gain access to a patient. (C 7-2.4)

    a. true
    b. false

18. Always remember to measure and place the proper size rigid type C-Collar onto the victim prior to placing the victim onto a short or long spine board. (C 7-2.4)

    a. true
    b. false

19. _____ is the process of preparing the patient to be moved from the scene of their accident or entrapment to the transport vehicle. (C 7-2.4)

    a. Preparation
    b. Transfer
    c. Packaging
    d. Extrication

20. The process of physically removing the injured patient from within the wreckage is known as the: (C 7-2.4)

    a. stabilization phase
    b. extrication phase
    c. triage phase
    d. transfer phase

Scenario

Read each scenario. Write the answers to the corresponding questions in the space provided.

SCENARIO #1:

You and your partner have returned to the station following a particularly stressful call involving a suspected child abuse victim. While you are debriefing, the radio sounds and you are instructed to respond to the scene of an automobile vs. truck accident. Dispatch informs you that reports have been received that three persons are trapped in the car. The truck driver is ambulatory at the scene.

continued

When you arrive at the scene, you find that two of the three victims in the automobile are still alive. One victim is exhibiting agonal respirations and trapped under the truck. The other entrapped victim is alert and oriented and is positioned such that extrication will not be difficult.

1. What is the first priority that you and your crew need to consider?

_____

_____

_____

_____

2. What initial steps should you take?

_____

_____

_____

_____

3. How will you handle this incident?

_____

_____

_____

_____

4. Which victims have the lowest priority during extrication?

_____

_____

_____

_____

CHAPTER 40 ANSWERS TO REVIEW QUESTIONS

1. a	5. c	9. d	13. a	17. a
2. a	6. b	10. d	14. d	18. a
3. a	7. a	11. c	15. c	19. c
4. a	8. b	12. a	16. d	20. b

SCENARIO SOLUTIONS

Scenario #1

1. Your first priority must be to determine that the scene is safe for you and your crew, as well as for other rescuers. You then size up the situation.

2. An assessment of the damage to the vehicles indicates that additional help will be needed. You instruct dispatch to send the needed assistance. It is also obvious that this situation will involve a complicated extrication process.

3. Since personal safety and scene size-up have been accomplished, you and your partner now move to the vehicles and begin the process of triage. Assign resources as they become available to extrication, patient care, and transport.

4. The obviously dead victim has the lowest priority during extrication. The patient who exhibited agonal respirations is also a low-priority transport.

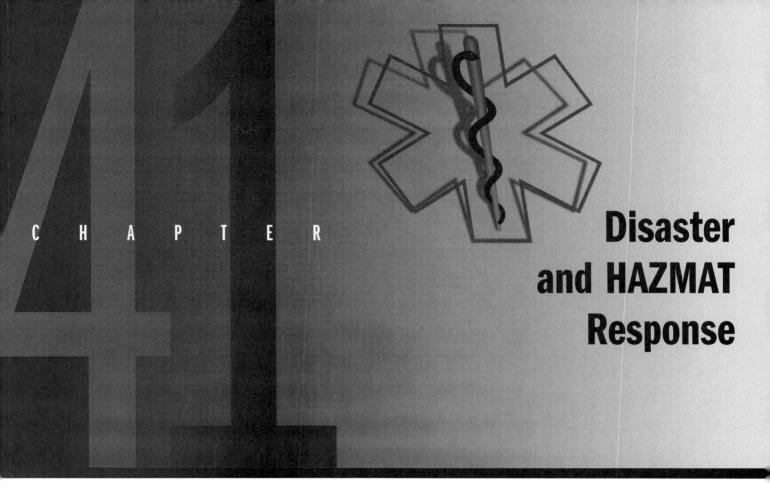

Disaster and HAZMAT Response

Reading Assignment: Chapter 41, pgs. 753–768

OBJECTIVES

1. Describe the characteristics of a disaster and differentiate these characteristics from normal operational conditions.

2. Identify the importance of disaster planning in disaster preparedness.

3. Explain the roles and responsibilities of the EMT in a disaster or multiple-casualty situation.

4. Demonstrate the ability to use the principles of triage in a multiple-casualty situation.

5. Define HAZMAT, and explain the significance for EMS operations.

6. Explain the federal regulations concerning HAZMAT training for emergency responders.

7. Review the rules for scene safety and identify the tools that are available to the EMT for managing a HAZMAT situation.

8. Describe the EMT's roles and responsibilities at a HAZMAT incident.

INTRODUCTION

This chapter deals with two types of infrequent incidents: disaster (or multiple-casualty situations) and HAZMAT. Emergency Medical Services systems and providers should be prepared to deal with these incidents when they occur. These situations often result in unusual types or numbers of injuries and require different methods of sorting, treating, and transporting patients. Disaster and HAZMAT responses present unique dangers to EMS providers.

The goal of this chapter is to provide the basic information necessary for the EMT to function effectively in these situations. Mastery of these topics requires specialized training and experience that exceed the boundaries of this text. Emergency medical technicians who will be involved in routine response to these specialized situations should complete additional specialized training.

REVIEW QUESTIONS

Please circle one correct answer for each question.

1. In general, an MCI exists when an incident has occurred that changes the normal ratio of rescuers and equipment to patients. (C 7-3.7)

   a. true
   b. false

2. Which of the following is not typical of all disasters? (C 7-3.11)

   a. road damage
   b. large numbers of injuries
   c. power outage
   d. housing damage

3. Examples of MCI include all of the following **except:** (C 7-3.7)

   a. a hurricane that strikes four states
   b. airplane crash
   c. bus accident
   d. an explosion in an apartment building

4. A two-car accident with four serious injuries in a remote rural community may be classified as a multiple casualty incident. (C 7-3.7)

   a. true
   b. false

5. Patients triaged as low priority include all of the following **except:** (C 7-3.9)

   a. minor, painful, swollen, deformed extremities
   b. minor, soft tissue injuries or death
   c. injuries incompatible with life
   d. burns or shock

6. Major components of MCI preplanning involve: (C 7-3.13)

   a. risk assessment
   b. resource identification
   c. practice
   d. all of the above

7. A list of resources for an MCI should include: (C 7-3.13)

   a. people
   b. equipment
   c. vehicles
   d. all of the above

8. Patients triaged as second priority include all of the following **except:** (C 7-3.9)

   a. back injuries with or without spinal cord damage
   b. heart attack or stroke
   c. burns without airway problems
   d. major or multiple bone or joint injuries

9. A comprehensive resource inventory identifies the resources available only inside of the local EMS system. (C 7-3.13)

   a. true
   b. false

10. Hazardous material incidents are dangerous for EMS providers because they require a different thought process and approach than do traditional EMS responses. (C 7-3.1)

    a. true
    b. false

11. In what order should the priorities be placed at a HAZMAT scene? (C 7-3.2 and C 7-3.3 and C 7-3.4)

    a. patient safety, EMT safety, bystander safety
    b. EMT safety, bystander safety, patient safety
    c. bystander safety, patient safety, EMT safety
    d. patient safety, bystander safety, EMT safety

12. Which of the following is not a high priority patient at an MCI (C 7-3.9)

    a. decreased mental status, severe burns
    b. uncontrolled or severe bleeding
    c. injuries incompatible with life
    d. airway and breathing difficulties

13. An EMT can prevent contamination to himself by doing which of the following? (C 7-3.12)

    a. decontamination of the transport vehicle
    b. remove and clean clothing
    c. vigorous handwashing
    d. all of the above

14. The EMT will usually be involved in doing detailed assignments within a sector and will rarely perform the role of sector commander. (C 7-3.10)

   ⓐ true
   b. false

15. Triage is the generic term used to describe: (C 7-3.9)

   a. vehicles used in a disaster response
   ⓑ systems of sorting or prioritizing patients
   c. EMS response levels
   d. the command sector at an MCI

16. When should the first-arriving EMS personnel start triage? (C 7-3.8)

   a. immediately upon arrival at the MCI
   b. when the all sectors have been established
   ⓒ as soon as scene safety has been assured
   d. as soon as all responding personnel have arrived

17. Contaminated patients may have to be treated in areas of the hospital other than the emergency department; therefore, advanced notification should be given to the receiving hospital. (Chp. Obj. #5)

   ⓐ true
   b. false

18. Patients who are still alive, but have wounds that are obviously fatal, are placed in the: (C 7-3.9)

   a. highest priority before patients in shock
   b. urgent priority before heart attack patients
   ⓒ lowest category immediately ahead of the dead.
   d. second priority after highest priority

19. The typical MCI plan calls for: (C 7-3.13)

   a. all high-priority patients to one hospital
   ⓑ matching the patients to the hospital's capabilities
   c. all low-priority patients to be transported first
   d. all second priority patients to be transported last

20. Which of the following contribute to the dangers for an EMT at a HAZMAT incident?

   a. lack of specific training in the management of HAZMAT incidents
   b. EMS providers are often the first emergency responders to arrive at the scene of an incident involving HAZMAT
   c. lack of protective equipment necessary to operate in a HAZMAT environment safely
   ⓓ all of the above

21. The first, key step in successfully managing a HAZMAT response is: (C 7-3.5)

   a. scene safety
   b. decontamination
   ⓒ recognition
   d. treatment

22. The U.S. Department of Transportation's *Emergency Response Handbook: Guidebook for Hazardous Materials Incidents:* (C 7-3.5)

    a. provides basic emergency information for known HAZMATs
    b. has information corresponding to the 4-digit number on a placard
    c. should be carried by every emergency response vehicle
    d. all of the above

23. At a HAZMAT incident, the EMS provider should wait until victims are extricated and decontaminated by HAZMAT specialists prior to starting any medical treatment. (C 7-3.12)

    a. true
    b. false

24. The ICS is a method for sorting and prioritizing patients.

    a. true
    b. false

25. In triage, it is absolutely critical that the EMT not become committed to a single patient until the overall sorting and prioritizing is accomplished. (C 7-3.9)

    a. true
    b. false

Scenario

Read each scenario. Write the answers to the corresponding questions in the space provided.

SCENARIO #1:

You and your partner are enjoying a quiet evening at the small rural ambulance service where you are working when a call comes in. The dispatcher directs you to a "three vehicle pile-up" on the nearby interstate. As you jump in the unit and prepare to respond, your conversation immediately turns to the probable availability of assistance on this one. You quickly recall that there are two receiving hospitals at your disposal—one hospital is located some 12 minutes away from the scene, while the other, larger facility is approximately 15 minutes away.

After arriving on the scene and completing the initial triage you determine that there are eight injured people. Your patient injury list reads as follows:

Patient #1: is entrapped in his vehicle and is exhibiting agonal respirations
Patient #2: is ambulatory with a painful, swollen, deformed extremity
Patient #3: was ejected from the vehicle, has obvious head injuries and is exhibiting posturing
Patient #4: has multiple lacerations and is complaining of glass in his eyes
Patient #5: has been pulled from the vehicle by a bystander and has obvious paradoxical respirations . . . this patient is conscious
Patient #6: has an open, painful, swollen, deformed area in his upper right leg
Patient #7: is crying that she cannot feel her legs
Patient #8: has burns on the left side of his torso from lying next to the exhaust pipe of his vehicle

As gasoline spills are obvious, fire units are also dispatched. The only extrication truck in your county is busy at another site and will not be available for a least another hour. Dispatch informs you that there are four other ambulance units available, all within 10 minutes of the scene.

continued

1. List, in correct sequence, the patient triage priorities.

   _____

   _____

   _____

2. List at least two scene hazards.

   _____

   _____

   _____

3. What are the considerations regarding patient transport and appropriate facilities?"

   _____

   _____

   _____

CHAPTER 41 ANSWERS TO REVIEW QUESTIONS

1. a	**6.** d	**11.** b	**16.** c	**21.** c
2. b	**7.** d	**12.** c	**17.** a	**22.** d
3. a	**8.** b	**13.** d	**18.** c	**23.** a
4. a	**9.** b	**14.** a	**19.** b	**24.** b
5. d	**10.** a	**15.** b	**20.** d	**25.** a

SCENARIO SOLUTIONS

Scenario #1:

1. The correct sequence for the patient triage priorities is as follows:

   - **Highest priority:** patient #3, patient #5
   - **Second priority:** patient #4, patient #6, patient #7, and patient #8
   - **Lowest Priority:** patient #1, patient #2

2. Scene hazards include gasoline spills, unstable vehicles, and traffic flow problems.

3. Considerations regarding patient transport and appropriate facilities include:

   - Call for backup from the other available ambulance units and, if available, aeromedical transport.
   - Determine which of the available facilities can accept the high-priority patients.
   - Determine the total number of patients that both hospitals can handle.
   - Understand that both high-priority patients should be transported to the facility with capabilities for definitive care.

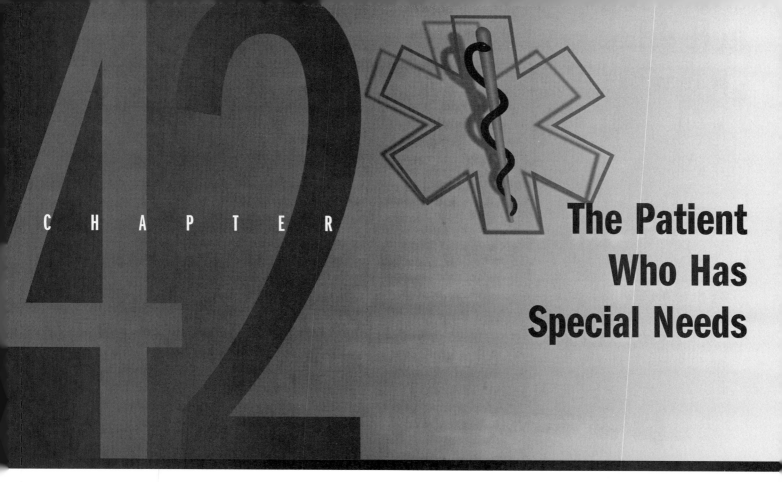

The Patient Who Has Special Needs

C H A P T E R **42**

Reading Assignment: Chapter 42, pgs. 769–785

OBJECTIVES

1. Discuss methods of providing care to patients who have special needs.

2. Identify developmental considerations for patients with special needs.

3. Describe examples of physical and developmental disabilities.

4. Identify feelings of the family and/or caregivers in relation to an ill or injured patient who has special needs.

5. Explain the need for knowledge and skills to treat patients who have special needs.

6. Discuss the provider's own emotional response to caring for a patient with special needs.

7. Develop methods of providing emergency care while appreciating the unique needs of each patient and family.

INTRODUCTION

The EMT-B is presented many instances wherein he or she must interact with and treat patients who have special needs. The purpose of this chapter is to give the EMT student the information to learn about this unique group before being called to treat them.

Myths and prejudices surround individuals who have disabilities. Many people tend to talk **about** a child who has mental retardation instead of talking **to** the child. Although it is imperative that the EMS provider understands the patient's disability, this chapter focuses on the importance of treating the illness or injury rather than the disability.

REVIEW QUESTIONS

Please circle one correct answer for each question.

1. All of the following are examples of developmental and physical disabilities **except:** (Chp. Obj. #3)

    a. Alzheimer's disease
    b. mental retardation
    c. cerebral palsy
    d. rubella

2. The term hemiplegia means paralysis on one half of the body. (Chp. Obj. #3)

    a. true
    b. false

3. All of the following are examples of chronic illness **except:** (Chp. Obj. #7)

    a. epilepsy
    b. myocardial infarction
    c. asthma
    d. renal failure

4. Asthma is the most common cause of school absences in children. (Chp. Obj. #3)

    a. true
    b. false

5. When dealing with a person who has special needs, life-threatening conditions should be treated before giving consideration to the disability. (Chp. Obj. #5)

    a. true
    b. false

6. The family of a disabled patient should be: (Chp. Obj. #4)

    a. respected
    b. involved in the patient's care in whatever way possible
    c. used as a resource and regarded as experts in their loved one's care
    d. all of the above

7. Special needs are conditions with the potential to interfere with usual growth and development. (Chp. Obj. #2)

    a. true
    b. false

8. Conditions with the potential to interfere with usual growth and development may involve all of the following **except:** (Chp. Obj. #3)

    a. physical disabilities, developmental disabilities
    b. chronic illnesses
    c. forms of technological support
    d. acute illnesses

9. Causes of developmental disabilities include all of the following **except:** (Chp. Obj. #3)

    a. metabolic disorders
    b. infections
    c. intracranial hemorrhage
    d. increased cerebral perfusion

10. Mental retardation is an example of a developmental disability. (Chp. Obj. #2)

    a. true
    b. false

11. Physical disabilities involve some type of limitation of mobility. (Chp. Obj. #2)

    a. true
    b. false

12. Causes of physical disabilities include: (Chp. Obj. #2)

    a. birth anomalies (i.e., spina bifida)
    b. head and spinal cord injuries
    c. infections resulting in paralysis (i.e., meningitis)
    d. all of the above

13. Cerebral palsy (CP) is a neuromuscular disability. Most people who have CP have a normal level of intelligence. (Chp. Obj. #1)

    a. true
    b. false

14. A person who has CP has difficulty controlling the voluntary muscles due to damage to a portion of the: (Chp. Obj. #3)

    a. brain
    b. spine
    c. liver
    d. heart

15. In individuals who have severe CP, swallowing may be compromised, which puts them at a higher risk for: (Chp. Obj. #5)

    a. kidney infections
    b. respiratory difficulties
    c. liver failure
    d. heart disease

16. In patients who have CP, airway obstruction can occur from increased secretions or food. (Chp. Obj. #5)

    a. true
    b. false

17. Spina bifida is the number one disabling birth anomaly in the United States. (Chp. Obj. #3)

    a. true
    b. false

18. Myelomeningocele, involving the meninges and the spinal cord, is the most serious form of spina bifida. (Chp. Obj. #3)

    a. true
    b. false

19. A common occurrence in spina bifida is the presence of hydrocephalus, in which: (Chp. Obj. #3)

    a. cerebrospinal fluid accumulates in the brain
    b. lifelong treatment may be required
    c. a shunt is inserted from the brain to another place in the body
    d. all of the above

20. Caregivers receive education about caring for specific equipment while in the hospital prior to discharge. They may: (Chp. Obj. #6)

    a. experience a great deal of anxiety until they become familiar with the equipment
    b. be very frightened if a malfunction occurs or the device does not operate as it did in the hospital
    c. call for assistance at the first sign of trouble, especially in the first few weeks of the adjustment phase
    d. all of the above

21. You should perform initial and ongoing assessments on individuals who have special needs using the same method as indicated for patients without these needs. (Chp. Obj. #1)

    a. true
    b. false

22. Many infants born prematurely use an apnea monitor at home to warn caregivers of any cessation of breathing. (Chp. Obj. #7)

    a. true
    b. false

23. When dealing with the special needs patient, pertinent questions that should be asked of the patient, parent, or caregiver include: (Chp. Obj. #7)

    a. "Does your child take medications for his or her seizures?"
    b. "What is different today that prompted you to call for an ambulance?"
    c. "Is your child able to take anything by mouth?"
    d. all of the above

24. To determine the patient's level of ability, the EMT should: (Chp. Obj. #5)

   a. talk with the patient, parent, or caregiver
   b. direct your questions in a positive light
   c. realize that the focus is on the patient's abilities instead of their disabilities
   d. all of the above

25. Many people who have physical disabilities use some type of adaptive device. These devices include: (Chp. Obj. #7)

   a. wheelchair
   b. braces
   c. crutches
   d. all of the above

Scenario

Read each scenario. Write the answers to the corresponding questions in the space provided.

SCENARIO #1:

You and your partner are called to the scene of a child having seizures. When you arrive on the scene, a teenage female is found lying in a bed. Her parents inform you that she has been deaf and mute since birth. She was just brought home from a Neuro unit in a nearby city.

Initial assessment reveals focal motor seizures. You note that the patient has a ventricular shunt in place. The patient's mother requests that you transfer the patient to the ER for further evaluation.

1. List at least four considerations regarding the care and management of this patient.

   _____

   _____

   _____

   _____

2. List four methods to involve the parents in the care of this patient.

   _____

   _____

   _____

   _____

3. What are the identified special needs for this patient?

   _____

   _____

   _____

   _____

CHAPTER 42 ANSWERS TO REVIEW QUESTIONS

1. d	**6.** d	**11.** a	**16.** a	**21.** a
2. a	**7.** a	**12.** d	**17.** a	**22.** a
3. b	**8.** d	**13.** a	**18.** a	**23.** d
4. a	**9.** d	**14.** a	**19.** a	**24.** d
5. a	**10.** a	**15.** b	**20.** d	**25.** d

SCENARIO SOLUTIONS

Scenario #1:

1. Considerations regarding the care and management of this patient include:

   - Airway.
   - Provide high-concentration oxygen.
   - Breathing.
   - Circulation.
   - Disability.
   - Attempt to gain more information about the child's history and any current health concerns.
   - Continue to reassess the child, and make contact with the receiving facility.
   - Document all assessment findings and interventions.
   - Throughout the call, talk softly to the child.
   - Try to limit the number of providers touching him.

2. Methods to involve the parent in the care of the patient include:

   - Allow them to stay with the child as much as possible as long as they are emotionally capable of doing so.
   - Allow the parents to function as your communication link to the patient.
   - Involve the parents in the patient's care in whatever way possible.
   - Use the parents as a resource and regard them as experts in their loved one's care.

3. Identified special needs for this patient include:

   - age
   - seizure precautions
   - shunt
   - communication